Group Activities *for* Latino/a Youth

Directly applicable to practice, *Group Activities for Latino/a Youth* allows helping professionals such as human service workers, social workers, and school and community mental health counselors to select and apply a series of group sessions with topics relevant to today's Latino/a youth. Each session contains detailed directions, and suggested discussion questions, with topic examples including grief, identity development, and conflict resolution. Sessions draw on Latino/a cultural norms and strengths to build culturally informed communication and coping skills in an effort to improve educational, social, and career outcomes. A developmental perspective is used, and sessions are designed to be creative and interactive to appeal to the high energy and playfulness of youth at any age. *Group Activities for Latino/a Youth* helps professionals to better engage and retain Latino/a clients, a group that traditionally experiences one of the largest dropout rates in therapy, often due to interventions largely informed by dominant Anglo norms and traditions.

Krista M. Malott, PhD is an associate professor at Villanova University. A licensed professional counselor, she has worked as a bilingual (Spanish-English) counselor with Latino youth and their families across a myriad of settings, including schools, a drug and alcohol clinic, a prison in Ecuador, and a domestic violence shelter.

Tina R. Paone, PhD is an associate professor at Monmouth University. A licensed professional counselor and registered play therapist supervisor, she incorporates the use of creative activities to teach about diversity topics in the classroom.

GROUP ACTIVITIES *for* LATINO/A YOUTH

STRENGTHENING IDENTITIES AND RESILIENCIES
THROUGH COUNSELING

EDITED BY

KRISTA M. MALOTT AND TINA R. PAONE

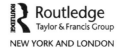
Routledge
Taylor & Francis Group

NEW YORK AND LONDON

First published 2016
by Routledge
711 Third Avenue, New York, NY 10017

and by Routledge
2 Park Square, Milton Park, Abingdon, Oxon, OX14 4RN

Routledge is an imprint of the Taylor & Francis Group, an informa business

© 2016 Taylor & Francis

Library of Congress Cataloging-in-Publication Data
A catalog record for this book has been requested

ISBN: 978-1-138-80678-8 (hbk)
ISBN: 978-1-138-80679-5 (pbk)
ISBN: 978-1-315-75148-1 (ebk)

Typeset in Garamond Three and Akzidenz Grotesk
by Swales & Willis Ltd, Exeter, Devon, UK

CONTENTS

....

CONTENTS

ILLUSTRATIONS

FIGURES

TABLE

EDITOR BIOGRAPHIES

Krista M. Malott, PhD, LPC began her career as a bilingual (Spanish-English) counselor, working with Spanish-speaking families and groups in various settings in North Carolina and Colorado, including school settings, a domestic violence shelter, and a drug and alcohol treatment center. She has since worked across populations in Ecuador and Guatemala, as a counselor and counselor educator. Currently, she is an associate professor in the Department of Education and Counseling at Villanova University, Villanova, Pennsylvania. In this role, she trains master's-level mental health counselors and undergraduate counseling minor students, with areas of instructional expertise including multicultural counseling, school counseling, and group counseling skills. In addition, she teaches in the undergraduate Intergroup Relations' program, which uses a small-group format to increase social justice through fostering relationships among people from different socioeconomic, gender, racial and ethnic groups. Her research emphasizes racial and ethnic identity development, with related topics of discrimination and effective multicultural counseling.

Tina R. Paone, PhD, LPC, RPT-S is an associate professor in the Department of Speech Pathology, Educational Counseling, and Leadership at Monmouth University, West Long Branch, New Jersey. In this role, she trains master's-level school counseling students in the areas of group counseling and advanced multicultural counseling. Her scholarly interests and research emphasize racial and ethnic identity development, group counseling, and play/activity therapy techniques. Additionally, she is the clinical director of the Counseling Center at Heritage, LLC in Montgomeryville, Pennsylvania where she provides therapy to youth and their families with specialty services in the areas of play therapy, racial and ethnic identity development, and transracial adoption. Prior to becoming a counselor educator, she worked in a variety of settings in Florida and Nevada including school settings, a rape crisis center, on a suicide crisis line, a domestic violence shelter, and a group home for girls on probation and parole.

CONTRIBUTORS

....

Dr. Katrina Cook is a counselor educator at Texas A&M University – San Antonio in San Antonio, Texas. She has worked in higher education since 2008. She has worked as a school counselor for 18 years and has also worked in the mental health field. She has experience working with adolescents, substance abuse, and expressive modalities.

Dr. Lisa M. Edwards is an associate professor in the department of Counselor Education and Counseling Psychology at Marquette University. In her current position, Dr. Edwards is the director of Counselor Education, directs the Culture and Well-Being Research Lab, and is a licensed psychologist in the state of Wisconsin. Dr. Edwards' research focuses on strengths and positive functioning among ethnic minority youth and adults.

Ijeoma Ezeofor, M.A., is a doctoral candidate in the Counseling Psychology program at the University of Maryland. She has co-facilitated several groups with adult clients, co-led group dialogues on issues of culture and privilege, and led educational programs for youth of color.

Dr. Tamara Hinojosa is a counselor educator at Texas A&M University – San Antonio in San Antonio, Texas. She has worked in higher education since 2004 and has worked in community mental health with a focus on academic advising, career counseling, women's issues, and crisis intervention counseling.

Dr. Kara Ieva is an assistant professor in the Counseling in Educational Settings program at Rowan University. She is a former Spanish teacher and school counselor in both the middle and high school settings. Currently, she is the principal investigator and project director for the Rowan University Aim High Science and Technology Academies that aids first-generation and low-income college students' access and preparation for postsecondary education.

Magnolia Kortland, NCC, M.Ed. & MSEd translated the session content of this book into Spanish. She is a graduate of the School Counseling program at Monmouth University. She has been a Spanish teacher at Old Bridge High School in New Jersey for the past 11 years and has a strong interest in multicultural counseling and a passion for helping youth experiencing marginalization.

Dr. José M. Maldonado is an associate professor of counseling at Monmouth University. He has over 15 years of professional experience as a mental health counselor, school counselor, and professor. As a clinician, he has worked extensively with a diversity of at-risk clientele and their families in urban environments. His research interests include multicultural counseling, family advocacy, and clinical supervision.

Dr. Mary G. Mayorga is a counselor educator at Texas A&M University – San Antonio in San Antonio, Texas. She has worked in higher education since 2005 and has worked extensively in the mental health field. She has experiences in different areas including grief work, adolescents, couples and family therapy, substance abuse, domestic violence, and sexual abuse.

Jessica B. McClintock, M.S. is a doctoral candidate in the Department of Counselor Education and Counseling Psychology at Marquette University. Her research focuses on uncovering strengths and building resilience as a means to foster well-being in diverse populations. Specifically, she explores how the positive psychology construct of hope and innate factors such as resilience promote positive functioning among African American youth and adults.

Dr. Suzanne Mudge is program coordinator for the counseling program at Texas A&M University – San Antonio in San Antonio, Texas. She has been a mental health professional for 28 years, a counselor supervisor for 12 years, and a counselor educator for 10 years. With an extensive background in school counseling, she is experienced working with children, adolescents, and families.

Dr. Pietro Sasso is an assistant professor of student affairs and college counseling at Monmouth University. With over a decade of experience in higher education and precollege bridge programs, he has worked across both secondary and postsecondary education. Dr. Sasso's research agenda is focused on identity construction and college student development outcomes.

Richard Q. Shin, PhD, is an associate professor in the Counseling, Higher Education, and Special Education department in the College of Education at the University of Maryland, College Park. He is the coordinator of the School Counseling program and holds an affiliate appointment in Counseling Psychology. He has taught group work throughout his career and specializes in scholarship related to social justice, discrimination, critical consciousness, and resiliency factors among youth of color.

Dr. Elizabeth A. Wardle is a counselor educator at Texas A&M University – Kingsville, in Kingsville, Texas. She has worked in higher education since 2007 and has extensive experience in the community mental health field, including working with HIV/AIDS patients and substance abuse. Dr. Wardle is also a Registered Nurse and has been able to use her nursing experience in the field of counseling.

Kristina Weiss is a K-8 school counselor in Berlin, New Jersey. She has extensive experience in facilitating groups with youth of all ages, from preschool to college level. Her expertise in group counseling ranges from grief and loss, sexual identity, social skills, and anxiety, to building relationships and friendships.

Jamie C. Welch, M.Ed., is a doctoral student in the Counseling Psychology program at the University of Maryland. He has experience facilitating group dialogues around social identity, power, oppression, and privilege in higher education settings.

INTRODUCTION

"I could go on and on about how it's so awesome to know more about our culture and share with others about it."

Juan, participant, ethnic identity group,
Mexican-origin youth, 2009

This book provides a collection of group activities with the ultimate goal of promoting the academic, career, and personal success of Latino/a youth. To appeal to youth, these sessions draw upon creative and expressive arts and contemporary issues. They are easily adapted for youth at different ages, and can be tailored for various ethnic and racial groups (e.g., Asians or Black/African Americans). However, to fill a void in the current literature regarding a large and expanding population across the United States, group sessions in this resource are premised on Latino/a cultural traditions and traits. Many of the sessions have been applied by the authors in group settings with Latino/a adolescents of various ages, and the experiences have been described by many of the youth as enjoyable, meaningful, and even life-changing. As written anonymously by one teen who participated in the Latino/a Youth and Ethnic Identity Development group of Chapter 4, "I learned [in group] that Latinos have worth and that we can get ahead and succeed."

Regardless of the ethnic or racial identities of the youth you choose to work with in applying these sessions, your status as an adult and group facilitator will mark you as the go-to expert regarding group goals, from strengthening ethnic identity to coping with the loss of a loved one. You will also likely be perceived as an expert on the group members themselves. For those reasons, in the next few chapters of this book, tenets of a very large and heterogeneous group identified beneath the umbrella term of *Latino/a* will be defined and described. Descriptors include history, demography, contributions, and cultural traits across the group. We recognize that fully and accurately describing such a diverse group is an impossible feat, considering the complexity and varied contributions of the many Latino/a subgroups, from Mexicans, to Puerto Ricans, to Colombians. Hence, readers may want to seek out additional readings and training experiences, if the Latino/a population is one that is new to them.

Specifically, Chapter 1 will attempt to describe Latino/as according to history, values, traits, and overall demographics. Chapter 2 will address challenges or barriers experienced by present-day Latino/a youth, to increase facilitator understanding of those issues that will undoubtedly surface during group sessions. Chapter 3 provides a framework for personal reflection of your own ethnic and racial identity, so that you can better facilitate such conversations with the youth you serve. Indeed, researchers have demonstrated the importance of helper self-knowledge and awareness regarding personal identity traits (as well as the willingness to acknowledge such) when working with clientele of color (Day-Vines et al., 2007). In addition, the premise of this book is that strong identities make for strong and successful human beings, with a vast ocean of research to support this, as will be discussed in the next few chapters. We believe this to be as equally true for clients as it is for those in the helper role—and the adult group facilitator can be a particularly influential role model in reflecting a strong and positive self-identity.

The remaining chapters of the book offer detailed outlines of various groups, each a set of six sessions. Topics are designed to address issues common to many of today's youth, such as grief, discrimination, communication skills, peer pressure, gender norms, goal setting, and exploring, understanding, and strengthening self-identity. Sessions were created to be low cost, with materials required that are easily obtainable. Many of the handouts used in the sessions are included, and efforts were made to provide materials in both Spanish and English. Most sessions can be used with small or large numbers of participants, although researchers have found that outcomes tend to be most positive with five to nine members (Burlingame, McClendon, & Alonso, 2011). Individual sessions can be pulled out and applied separately or used in sequence. Some, such as the *Creando Esperanza: Hope Groups* sessions of Chapter 7, were designed to build upon one another.

Finally, a note about the terminology applied across this book. We recognize Latino/a as an umbrella term that includes myriad subgroups with diverse traits and origins, from Mayan descendants of Guatemalan origin who speak neither English nor Spanish, to blond-haired Argentines who practice Judaism and speak German. Research tells us that most Latino/a individuals prefer to be addressed and understood uniquely, according to personal label preferences (Malott, 2009; Zarate, Bhimji, & Reece, 2005). Preferences and meanings of assumed ethnic labels can change for individuals according to development, settings, and situations. However, *Latino/a* will be applied throughout this book to represent the many subgroups, to honor use of that terminology by current scholars and demographers, and in response to the expressed preferences of many Latino/as in our and others' research who have eschewed *Hispanic* as a governmentally imposed, and therefore less desirable, term (Malott, 2009; Therrien & Ramirez, 2000). Finally, the use of both the feminine 'a' and the masculine 'o' at the end of the term *Latin* across the book offers a more gender-inclusive version of the traditionally used label, Latino.

REFERENCES

Burlingame, G. M., McClendon, D. T., & Alonso, J. (2011). Cohesion in group therapy. *Psychotherapy, 48*, 34–42. doi:10.1037/a0022063

Day-Vines, N. L., Wood, S. M., Grothaus, T., Craigen, L., Holman, A., Dotson-Blake, K., & Douglass, M. J. (2007). Broaching the subjects of race, ethnicity, and culture during the counseling process. *Journal of Counseling and Development, 85*, 401–409. doi:10.1002/j.1556-6678.2007.tb00608.x

Malott, K. M. (2009). Investigation of ethnic self-labeling in the Latina population: Implications for counselors and counselor educators. *Journal of Counseling & Development, 87*, 179–185. doi:10.1002/j.1556-6678.2009.tb00565.x

Therrien, M., & Ramirez, R. R. (2000). *The Hispanic population in the United States: March 2000 (Current Population Reports*, pp. 250–535). Washington, D.C.: U.S. Census Bureau. Retrieved from http://www.census.gov/prod/2001pubs/p20-535.pdf

Zarate, M. E., Bhimji, F., & Reece, L. (2005). Ethnic identity and academic achievement among Latino/a adolescents. *Journal of Latino/as and Education, 4*, 95–114. doi:10.1207/s1532771xjle0402_3

WHO ARE LATINO/AS?

Krista M. Malott and Tina R. Paone

Our parents grew up watching la India Maria
We grow up watching Family Guy
They ate tacos and tortas
While we eat hot dogs and hamburgers
They went to the plaza
While we go to the mall
Yet we still share some things in common
Like the language we speak
And our pride of being Mexican
                   Pennsylvanian Latino/a teens of Mexican descent, 2009

The question, *who are Latino/as*, could fill an entire library. However, to the best of our abilities, we will attempt to present an accurate description of such a diverse group, with particular trends and varied histories, with brevity in mind. Numbered at 53 million and comprising 17% of the total U.S. population, Latino/as are the largest population of color in the nation (U.S. Census, 2012a). It is predicted that the population will continue to rapidly expand, and that by 2060 Latino/as will comprise 31% of the entire population (approximately one out of every three individuals) (U.S. Census, 2008). This group is one of the fastest growing, in part due to high birth rates. For instance, over one out of four of all births (26.3%) across the nation in 2011 were to Latina women (Pew Hispanic Center, 2012). As a result, this is a young population, whereby nearly one out of three (33.8%) of all Latino/as is aged 18 or below, compared to 24% of the entire U.S. population (U.S. Census Bureau, 2012a). In fact, it is predicted that by 2020 Latino/as will comprise nearly one out of four of all U.S. youth in school (U.S. Hispanic Chamber of Commerce, 2007).

Considering subgroup trends, numbers show that 65% of Latino/as are of Mexican origin. Puerto Ricans are the next largest group (equaling 9.4% of all Latino/as), followed by Cubans (3.8%), Salvadorans (3.6%), Dominicans (3.0%), and Guatemalans (2.3%). The remaining percentage includes Latino/as of South or Central America or other origins (U.S. Census Bureau, 2013).

Although some Latino/as are descendants of ancestors who lived on the North American continent long before it became the United States, approximately 36% of all Latino/as are foreign born, with those numbers on the rise (Puerto Ricans excluded). Foreign-born Latino/as comprise over half (53.3%) of the total foreign-born population in the U.S (Pew Hispanic Center, 2013). Issues related to resources (work and health care) and naturalization are high for those who have recently arrived to the country, as Latino/as possess the lowest rate of naturalization of all foreign-born individuals (34.2% for those from South America, and 25% for Mexicans; U.S. Census Bureau, 2010; 2012b).

Latino/as can be found anywhere in the country, although larger concentrations have settled near entry ports to the nation (e.g., southern states close to the Mexican border) or urban areas where greater job opportunities exist. For instance, more than half of Latino/as live in Florida, California, and Texas, and the largest concentration of Latino/as (4.8 million) live in the Los Angeles region (U.S. Census Bureau, 2013). Sixteen other states in various regions of the country are home to at least a half-million Latino/a individuals each, with Latino/as frequently migrating to certain locations to be close to family members or job opportunities (U.S. Census Bureau, 2011).

A large portion of Latino/as speak Spanish, albeit of various dialects and with differing accents and vocabularies (and differing meanings for the same words). Spanish speakers comprise 12.9% of all U.S. residents, with 78% of all Latino/as indicating that they speak Spanish at home (U.S. Census Bureau, 2011). Youth from this population encompass the largest percentage of English language learners in the U.S. school system. For instance, of the 4.7 million limited English-proficient students identified in K-12 schools, 73% were Spanish speakers (Education Commission of the States, 2013).

Latino/as are a racially and ethnically diverse people, encompassing indigenous groups (two examples include Mayan and Inca), descendants of African slaves, and those of Spanish and other European heritage. As a result, the term *Mestizo* has been applied to indicate Latino/as with a blended ancestry of Spanish, indigenous, and African origins (Santiago-Rivera, Arredondo, & Gallardo-Cooper, 2002). In smaller numbers are the Latino/as of Middle Eastern and Asian descent. In the 2010 census, Latino/as were the population most likely to identify with multiple racial categories, with 1.9 million identifying as Black or multiracial. Considering specific racial identification, some choose to self-describe as White, while others classify themselves as Brown, Black, or simply *of color*. Similar to ethnic label choice, preferred racial labels will vary individually.

Black Latino/as will often claim a heritage and culture that is distinct from non-Hispanic African Americans, although others may mistake the two groups as one and the same. In addition, there is great diversity within the Black Latino/a population. For example, dark-skinned Cuban Americans (or self-described *Afro-Cubanos*) may perceive themselves as culturally different from Mexicans or Dominicans of similar skin tones. They and their family members will possess unique cultural practices, traditions, histories, and understandings of historical and contemporary racism, which in turn inform their beliefs about their own race (and racial labels). Such differences may result in conflict across Latino/a subgroups (Uhlmann, Dasgupta, Elgueta, Greenwalkd, & Swanson, 2002), while common experiences of racial discrimination within the U.S. can lead to shared struggles across subgroups—all factors that can be meaningfully explored in counseling groups (Malott, 2010).

SHARED VALUES AND TRADITIONS

Values and traditions of Latino/as will vary according to context and traits, including a person's origins, generational status, sociopolitical orientation, level of education, or acculturation status (e.g., the extent to which they have adopted dominant, U.S. cultural traits; McNeill, Prieto, Niemann, Pizarro, Vera, & Gómez, 2001). However, the majority of Latin American countries share a history of Spanish colonization, which has united many Latino/as across nations through a shared struggle for independence, as well as imparting defining traits such as the Spanish language and the Roman Catholic religion .

As a result, the majority of Latino/as share Roman Catholicism as their religion (approximately 80%), albeit blended, at times, with customs or traditions from indigenous (e.g., curanderos, or traditional healers) or African populations (e.g., voodoo, Santería). However, pockets of Latin America have also been home to refugees of various religions (e.g., Jewish, Muslim, Hindu, and Confucianism), which they then bring from Latin America to the U.S. Religion continues to be an important part of life for many Latino/as in the U.S., and prayer, as well as religious faith, can provide a form of spiritual support and value-informed guidance (Santiago-Rivera et al., 2002).

Shared traditional values for Latino/as are many and include *familismo* (the central role of family), *respeto* (respect), *personalismo* (the central role of personal relationships), *simpatía* (the maintenance of dignified and respectful social interactions), and *marianismo/machismo* (traditional gender roles for women and men; Arredondo et al., 2006). There is also a preference for hierarchical structure in relationships, reflected in the honoring of elders, male household figures, and those in positions of respect, such as teachers (Kanel, 2002).

Within Latino/a culture, values and morals are often shared across generations through proverbs or stories (*dichos* or *cuentos*). As such, they can be seen as tools used to transmit familial and societal values and norms (Arredondo et al., 2006). Examples of *dichos* that teach values follow, some of which have been incorporated into Chapter 4's sessions of this book:

- *No se le puede pedir peras al olmo* (you cannot ask an elm tree to bear pears). Value expressed: we should have realistic expectations.
- *El quien no habla, dios no lo oye* (if one does not speak out, God cannot listen). Value expressed: one must express oneself; if we want to find help, first we should do something for ourselves.
- *Una gota de agua puede labrar una piedra* (a drop of water can carve a rock). Value expressed: persistence can lead to achievement.
- *Agua que no has de beber, déjala correr* (water that you do not drink, let it run). Value expressed: Do not meddle in others' business.
- *Haz bien y no mires a quien* (do good unto others and look not to whom). Value expressed: do good deeds.

In addition to the oral tradition of transmitting values, Latino/as practice additional traditions. Food itself is historically and regionally distinct, with specialty dishes differing even from town to town. Across Latino/a cultures there is a general importance of sharing meals with families and friends. In fact, sharing of food within group sessions can offer a powerful means for joining and building trust. Geographic-specific examples of food traditions include sharing the Argentine tea, *yerba mate*, with friends and family members, cooking and eating a Guatemalan meal called *fiambre* during the Day of the Dead celebration in November of each year, or making tamales, an elaborate meat and cornmeal dish, in nearly any Latin American country during the holidays. Other traditions or celebrations that can be found across Latino/a cultures that continue to be practiced by many who have immigrated to the U.S. include *quinceañeras* (a coming-of-age celebration for girls turning 15), celebrations related to Christian holidays and venerated Saints, and recognition, remembrance, and celebration of loved ones who have died, dubbed All Souls Day and, somewhat related, for Mexicans, *Día de los Muertos*, or Day of the Dead (Menard, 2000).

HISTORY

Latino/as have resided on what is currently the United States long before the existence of the nation itself. Following a war with Mexico in 1848, the U.S. government annexed Western territories originally belonging to Mexico and, at one point, Spain. The majority of those Spanish-speaking residents (approximately 75,000) chose to stay in the U.S., becoming the first generation of Mexican Americans. Hence, Latino/as of Mexican origins, including many indigenous persons and Mestizos (those of Spanish-indigenous heritage), boast one of the longest residencies in the U.S. territory (Gutiérrez, 2004).

Shortly after the U.S.–Mexican war, Latino/as of other origins began migrating to the country. This migration was largely in response to existing (and growing) economic disparities between Latin American countries and the U.S. and, also, in relation to the U.S.'s economic, political, and military involvement in Latin America (Colby, 2013). Hence, Latino/as who have emigrated may bring with them conflicted perspectives and experiences related to U.S. presence and politics in their home countries. In an example of this, Guatemalan Mayans have fled their country as refugees over the past decades in part due to U.S. influence, which entailed U.S. involvement in a Guatemalan presidency that sparked a civil war and extreme violence toward the indigenous population. The U.S. government, in turn, has refused many Guatemalans refuge in the U.S., refuting the genocidal actions toward those individuals due to an investment in that nation's businesses and government (Colby, 2013; Coutin, 1993).

Puerto Ricans constitute a group with a unique history in the U.S., with individuals granted U.S. citizenship following acquisition of the island as a result of the Spanish-American War of 1898. In turn, Puerto Ricans have migrated to the United States in significant numbers, to become the second largest Latino/a subpopulation on the U.S. mainland. The country itself is considered a commonwealth, rather than a state of the United States; a status that prohibits voting representation within the Congress. Some from the commonwealth argue for making Puerto Rico a state, with full voting capabilities, while others continue to strive toward complete independence from the U.S. (Wagenheim & Jiménez de Wagenheim, 2013).

Hence, across U.S. history, from the 20th century to the present day, Latino/a migration has increased in number to surpass that of any other subpopulation in the country (Gutiérrez, 2004). Each individual brings a unique history according to his or her migration story, from hardships such as poverty or civil war, to the desire for adventure or economic and educational opportunities. Their stories are shaped by an additionally complex history of the (sometimes) exploitative relationship between U.S. governmental and economic policies and the Latino/a immigrant community. For instance, early in U.S. history, many Mexican Americans experienced a loss of rights to their lands, farms, or jobs as a result of discriminatory laws similar to *Jim Crow*. Such laws were meant to restrict their access to job and educational opportunities, relegating Latino/as to manual labor or service-type work. Those policies followed, and affected, Latino/as well into the 20th century (Gutiérrez, 2004).

Discrimination has not, however, deterred migrants from entering the country and working hard to contribute to its economy. Latino/as continuously sought to move beyond the restrictions imposed by individual and systematic exploitation and discrimination. Large changes came with the Civil Rights movement of the 1960s and 1970s, whereby Latino/as united in an effort to eradicate discrimination and achieve legal and social equality. It was at that time that the ethnic label, *Chicano*, was adopted by some Mexican Americans as a politicized label, to recognize ethnic pride and the struggle to achieve social and political equality. *Chicano* political activism also emerged as a new and, at times, militant form of political activism (Gutiérrez, 2004).

There were many historical figures who fought for the equal rights of Latino/as during that era and who could be meaningfully referenced as role models in group work with Latino/a youth. Some of the more well-known persons include Cesar Chavez, Rodolfo "Corky" Gonzales, Alurista (or Alberto Baltazar Urista Heredia), Reies López Tijerina, Dr. Hector P. Garcia, and Dolores Huera. Their own, and others', efforts resulted in many changes, including passage of voting rights legislation, the establishment of bilingual educational programs in schools, and the foundation in higher education of Latino/a studies. Emerging from that era were many powerful lobbying groups that exist to the present day, such as the National Council of La Raza, the League of United Latin American Citizens, and the Mexican

American Legal Defense and Education Fund (Gutiérrez, 2004). Such groups continue to fight for equality and access to resources for Latino/as across the nation.

CONTRIBUTION

Sociologist Curry Rodríguez (1999) surmised that "The United States has continuously benefitted from the contributions of immigrants, whether in terms of the seemingly mundane food on our tables, the care of our children, or the intellectual discoveries and musical contributions borne of the hands of our newer residents" (p. 70). Nowhere are Latino/as' contributions more apparent than in the country's economic sector. This is true regarding both entrepreneurship and consumerism.

Latino/as are the group most likely to start their own business, and Latino/a businessmen and women have assumed a vital and ever-increasing role in the U.S. economy. For instance, between 1997 and 2002, the growth rate of Latino/a-owned businesses (31%) was triple that of all business (10%). A 2013 report indicated more than 3.1 million businesses are owned by Latino/a individuals, contributing $468 billion to the U.S. economy annually (Geoscape, 2013). Latino/a consumers are also estimated to consume $1.2 trillion per year (Llopis, 2012).

The inception of the 21st century has seen Latino/as in every professional role. Indeed, this book itself is filled with the citations of prominent Latino/a scholars who have contributed significantly to the intellectual and educational endeavors of fellow scholars and learners alike. Politically, although there has yet to be a President of Latino/a heritage, 2009 was particularly meaningful in that Sonia Sotomayor was appointed as the country's first Latina Supreme Court justice. The growth of Latino/as over time has influenced politics itself, with the population's vote putting many persons of Latino/a heritage in varied prominent offices. In addition, a large and growing pool of Latino/a voters frequently incurs the wooing of non-Latino/a running candidates (note President Barack Obama's attempt to reach out to Mexican Americans during his 2008 campaign by singing the popular song, *Mexico Lindo*, in Spanish on a Mexican-America radio show in California).

Latino/as of all origins have enriched the United States according to language use, food choice, the performing arts, and literature (Ybarra-Frausto, n.d.). Artistic influences from Latino/a cultures include salsa dancing, with its origins in Afro-Caribbean dances, and myriad other musical genres, from

Afro-Cuban jazz to the more recent Panamanian-Puerto Rican-inspired *reggaeton*. Many contemporary artists have 'crossed over' and become popular figures in the dominant American public media, attesting to their broad appeal across groups. Examples of such figures include writers Alejandro Murguía, Junot Díaz, Sandra Cisneros, and Ray Gonzalez, musician and composer José Feliciano, and singers Ricky Martin and the late Selena.

Yet in spite of the many positive advancements and successes of present-day Latino/as, discriminatory barriers continue to exist today, albeit at a lesser intensity than decades before. For this reason, the historical struggles and triumphs experienced by Latino/as in the past are important to share with today's Latino/a adolescents. Youth need to learn of those figures who overcame, and currently are overcoming, great adversity, to provide models of inspiration in facing current barriers and stressors.

REFERENCES

Arredondo, P., Davison Avilés, R. M., Zalaquett, C. P., Grazioso, M. P., Bordes, V., Hita, L., & Lopez, B. (2006). The psychohistorical approach in family counseling with Mestizo/Latino/a immigrants: A continuum and synergy of worldviews. *The Family Journal, 14*, 13–27. doi:10.1177/1066480705283089

Colby, J. M. (2013). *The business of empire: United Fruit, race, and U.S. expansion in Central America (the United States in the world)*. Cornell, NY: Cornell University Press.

Coutin, S. B. (1993). *The culture of protest: Religious activism and the U.S. sanctuary movement*. Boulder, CO: Westview Press.

Curry Rodríguez, J. E. (1999). Immigrant contributions: Las contribuciones de los emigrantes. In J. Olmos, L. Ybarra, & M. Monterrey (eds.), *Americanos: Latino/a life in the United States La Vida Latina en los Estados Unidos* (pp. 70–83). New York, NY: Little, Brown and Company.

Education Commission of the States (2013). *English language learners: A growing—yet underserved—population*. Retrieved from www.ecs.org/per

Geoscape (2013). *Hispanic businesses and entrepreneurs drive growth in the new economy: 2013 report*. Retrieved from www.geoscape.com

Gutiérrez, D. G. (Ed.). (2004). *The Colombia history of Latino/as in the United States since 1960*. New York, NY: Colombia University Press.

Kanel, K. (2002). Mental health needs of Spanish-speaking Latino/as in southern California. *Hispanic Journal of Behavioral Sciences, 24*, 74–92. doi:10.1177/0739986302024001005

Llopis, G. (April 2012). *Earn the trust of Hispanic consumers and your brand will dominate.* Retrieved from http://www.forbes.com/sites/glennllopis/2012/04/02/earn-the-trust-of-hispanic-consumers-and-your-brand-will-dominate/

Malott, K. M. (2010). Being Mexican: Strengths and challenges of Mexican-origin adolescents. *Journal of School Counseling, 8*(12). Retrieved from http://jsc.montana.edu/

McNeill, B. W., Prieto, L. R., Niemann, Y. F., Pizarro, M., Vera, E. M., & Gómez, S. P. (2001). Current directions in Chicano/o psychology. *The Counseling Psychologist, 29*, 5–17. doi:10.1177/0011000001291001

Menard, V. (2000). *Latino holiday book: From Cinco de Mayo to Día de los Muertos—the celebrations and traditions of Hispanic Americans.* New York, NY: Marlowe & Company.

Pew Hispanic Center (2012). *Explaining why minority births now outnumber White births.* Retrieved from http://www.pewsocialtrends.org/2012/05/17/explaining-why-minority-births-now-outnumber-white-births/

Pew Hispanic Center (2013). *Hispanic population trends.* Retrieved from http://www.pewhispanic.org/2013/02/15/hispanic-population-trends/ph_13-01-23_ss_hispanics4/

Santiago-Rivera, A. L., Arredondo, P., & Gallardo-Cooper, M. (2002). *Counseling Latino and la familia: A practical guide.* Thousand Oaks, CA: Sage Publications.

Uhlmann, E., Dasgupta, N., Elgueta, A., Greenwald, A. G., & Swanson, J. (2002). Subgroup prejudice based on skin color among Hispanics in the United States and Latin America. *Social Cognition, 20*(3), 198–225. doi:10.1521/soco.20.3.198.21104

U.S. Census Bureau (2010). *The foreign-born population in the United States: 2010.* Retrieved from http://www.census.gov/population/foreign/

U.S. Census Bureau (2011). *Language spoken at home: 2011 American community survey 1-year estimates.* Retrieved from http://www.census.gov/hhes/socdemo/language/data/acs/

U.S. Census Bureau (2012a). *The Hispanic population in the United States: 2012.* Retrieved from https://www.census.gov/population/hispanic/data/2012.html

U.S. Census Bureau (2012b). *The Hispanic population in the United States: 2012.* Retrieved from https://www.census.gov/population/hispanic/data/2012.html

U.S. Census Bureau (2013). *Hispanic heritage month 2007: Sep 15-Oct. 15.* http://www.census.gov/newsroom/releases/archives/facts_for_features_special_editions/cb13-ff19.html

U.S. Hispanic Chamber of Commerce (2007). *Statistics: Population and economic strength*. Retrieved from http://www.ushcc.com/ res-statistics.html

Wagenheim, K., & Jiménez de Wagenheim, O. (2013). *The Puerto Ricans*. Princeton, NJ: Marcus Wiener Publishers.

Ybarra-Frausto, T. (n.d.). *A panorama of Latino arts*. National Park System Advisory Board. Retrieved from http://www.nps.gov/Latino/Latino/athemestudy/pdfs/Arts_FINAL_Web.pdf

STRESSORS AND BARRIERS FOR LATINO/A YOUTH

Krista M. Malott and Tina R. Paone

{Teachers} all expect you to do bad in classes, and they don't pay attention to you because they all think you're going to fail anyway.
                                        Juan, 16, Mexican American

Childhood and adolescence can be a stressful time of life for persons of any ethnicity. Adolescence is a particularly vulnerable period, characterized by major life and developmental changes and transitions (Ozer et al., 2011). In particular, teens must learn to balance a desire for independence with the simultaneous need for emotional and economic support. Across various Latino/a subgroups, youth may experience stressors that are both similar to, and distinct from, one another.

For instance, a third-generation, English-speaking, middle-class adolescent with blond hair and Argentinean roots will experience a set of challenges unique from a dark-skinned youth of Nicaraguan origins who recently entered the U.S. illegally, is living in poverty, and is just beginning to learn English. As a matter of fact, if asked, those two would likely agree that their daily experiences are about as different as two experiences can come. With this in mind, the following is a review of the many environmental stressors experienced by Latino/a youth, with commentary, when available in the data, on differences across subgroups (e.g., youth of Mexican origin, Cuban origin, etc.). Such issues will most certainly surface for youth as they participate in group sessions. Ideally, facilitators will be comfortable with exploring such concerns as they emerge. Group is most significant when it is both culturally *and* contextually relevant.

STRESSORS AND BARRIERS DEFINED

Educational Attainment

In spite of the fact that many Latino/as earn college degrees and obtain prestigious professional positions, statistics related to Latino/a school completion are the lowest of all groups. According to a 2013 report by the National Center for Education Statistics, 75% of Latino/as aged 25 to 29 had completed high school, compared to 96% for Asians, 95% for White non-Latino/as, and 89% for Blacks. At the college level, differences across groups seem to persist, with only 15% of Latino/as aged 25 to 29 having earned a bachelor's degree, compared to 62% of Asians, 40% Whites, and 23% Blacks (National Center for Education Statistics, 2013).

Across Latino/a subpopulations, differences in school attainment exist. For instance, 79% of Latino/as who emigrated to the U.S. during their lifetimes have attained a high school diploma, compared to 90% for second-generation Latino/as (U.S. Department of Education, 2012). Factors impeding school completion vary, with many first-generation youth citing the pressure to work and support family as one (The College Board Advocacy and Policy Center, 2010; Pew Hispanic Center, 2005). However, the following additional environmental stressors, experienced by Latino/as of various generations, have also been noted as factors for some in high school dropout.

Poverty and its Consequences

The 2000 Census showed that Latino/as without legal status were much more susceptible to unemployment or were employed in lower-paying service jobs. In turn, nearly one out of three Latino/as live in homes with incomes that are below the poverty line (The Annie E. Casey Foundation, 2014; Therrien & Ramirez, 2000). Differences exist across ethnic subgroups. Descendants of Spain, Cuba, and South America are more likely to live above the poverty line, while those with roots in Mexico, Central America, and the Caribbean more often live in poverty (The Annie E. Casey Foundation, 2014). Differential rates may in part have to do with the level of education, or socioeconomic status, immigrants achieved while in their home country.

In turn, researchers have cited a multitude of negative consequences related to living in poverty and in impoverished settings. Several of those include: (a) elevated levels of stress and anxiety, dubbed "toxic stress" (p. 3) by scholars (The Annie E. Casey Foundation, 2014) due to the effects of poverty on one's physical health, ability to concentrate and learn in school, and social mobility (Caughy, O'Campo, & Muntaner, 2003; Sapolsky, 2005); (b) increased stress and anxiety due to the continuous threat of neighborhood violence; (c) limited job and mentoring opportunities (Vega & Gil, 1999); (d) limited or no access to quality early childhood education, health, and mental health care; and (e) segregated, under-resourced neighborhoods (The Annie E. Casey Foundation, 2014; Pew Hispanic Center, 2004).

Poverty-related segregation has dramatic and negative impacts on students' academic and career achievement. Schools in segregated, impoverished neighborhoods are funded with local tax dollars and so are grossly under-resourced, in spite of the fact that many youth in those settings have greater needs due to poverty-related stressors. Those schools have been shown to experience multiple deficits, including: (a) the largest number of inexperienced and untrained teachers, as compared to better-funded schools with less-stressed populations (Davis & Welcher, 2013); (b) limited counseling and educational resources, and higher-stressed teachers who receive lower pay and inadequate support (National Commission on Teaching and America's Future, 2003); (c) larger class sizes; and (d) higher rates of teacher attrition (40–50%), which in turn reduces environmental stability and student mentoring and support (Darling-Hammond, 2004).

Additionally, Latino/a youth who live in poverty experience a double burden of lowered teacher, counselor, and administrator expectations, due to those professionals' often unconscious views of 'minority' and 'poor' youth as less capable. Such prejudices can result in deemphasizing learning over rote memorization and they have inspired zero-tolerance discipline policies that inadvertently serve to push students out of the schools and into the legal system (Tuck, 2012). The impact of such prejudices extends beyond academics, as one high-achieving Latina youth in a study (Malott, 2010) described her reaction to lowered teacher expectations: "I was very hurt because [they] thought that I was not good enough or that I couldn't do it" (p. 17). It should be of no surprise, then, that youth in such schools experience higher rates of dropout. Indeed, scholars have even suggested that school dropout from extremely underfunded and biased systems may actually be a better solution for youth, considering the often poor learning quality in the settings, along with the discriminatory treatment students of color experience (Tuck, 2012).

Finally, researchers and mental health experts have come to understand that living in poverty can induce a variety of behaviors in children that are viewed as defiant or disruptive to adults in school settings. Bloom (2005) noted these as trauma-induced behaviors for youth living in poverty, with grief responses as particularly salient for those who have experienced traumatic losses. Those living in poverty can suffer the loss of physical and psychological safety, and of friends, family members, and whole communities due to frequent geographical moves, violent deaths, or illnesses left untreated due to monetary issues (Bloom, 2005; Hopper, Bassuk, & Olivet, 2010). Poverty-related trauma and stress reactions can also mimic a variety of disorders, such as hyperactivity or conduct disorder. Such behaviors are frequently misunderstood, misdiagnosed, and, in turn, inappropriately treated with medication (Jacobson, 2014).

Career and Educational Planning and Mentoring

Youth who have the opportunity to explore and clarify career and educational goals with at least one adult in their lives are more likely to achieve greater educational and work success (Baum & Flores, 2011). However, youth of color, males in particular, have noted a dearth of supportive adults to initiate such conversations (The College Board Advocacy and Policy Center, 2010). Underfunded, under-resourced schools are less able to offer such guidance (Bryan, Moore-Thomas, Day-Vines, & Holcomb-McCoy, 2011). In turn, possibly due to a lack of adult guidance in college and career decision making, the majority of high-achieving youth who live in poverty do not apply to selective colleges, missing out on those institutions' "generous academic resources, increased financial aid, and better collegiate and career opportunities" (Hoxby & Turner, 2013, p. 2).

However, achievement of a college education is of strong value for many Latino/a families, and this value is reflected in a rate of college enrollment for Latino/as that recently surpassed that of Whites (Fry & Taylor, 2013). Indeed, Latino/as are the largest ethnic minority group on college campuses (Pew Hispanic Center, 2012). Over 40% of all Latino/as are first-generation college goers (Moreno, 2012), and many of those youth, unaware of other options, choose to attend undersourced community colleges, where they are more likely to be working and less likely to be knowledgeable of campus-wide support services (Bernal, Alemán, & Garavito, 2010). Latino/a youth attending four-year institutions more often accumulate large amounts of student debt (Policy Link, 2011), leaving them at a disadvantage in comparison to those receiving adult guidance in selecting schools that offer scholarships and support specific to youth of color (Greenstone & Looney, 2013).

In turn, college dropout rates are extremely high for Latino/as (51%) in comparison to Whites (40%) (Gonzalez, 2010). Reasons for college dropout largely relate to monetary issues and family obligations (The College Board Advocacy and Policy Center, 2010). However, additional, commonly cited reasons include discrimination related to social class, race, and ethnicity, and poor academic preparation, coupled with a lack of understanding in how to maneuver the system in finding academic and social support (Bernal et al., 2010; The College Board Advocacy and Policy Center, 2010; Harvard Graduate School of Education, 2011). Examples of survival skills that many first-generation college students may not have learned include ways to obtain tutoring assistance, community and campus clubs and resources, job and additional scholarship information, same-ethnic/race mentoring, and understanding norms in approaching university professors to ask for help (Bernal et al., 2010).

Language Barriers

For immigrants, the most important tool for success is the English language. The greatest barrier to learning English is the dearth of high-quality and affordable community or school-based language programs. Students in schools with language programs may experience discrimination or inappropriate placement related to their language skills, such as teacher and counselor misperception of language deficiency as a learning disability or low cognitive abilities. Another challenge is that many adults lack understanding of the fact that it takes time to learn a language: up to five years or 10,000 hours (Eaton, 2011). Conversely, Latino/a youth who are not recent immigrants and who are entirely fluent in English may be misperceived by teachers or potential employers as English impaired—a discriminatory experience noted by many of the youth we interviewed in one particular area of the Northeastern U.S. (Malott, 2010).

Teen Pregnancy

The good news is that teen birth rates have decreased for all groups in the past years. The rate of pregnancy for Latinas, ages 15–19, has dropped 34% from 2007 to 2011. In spite of this positive trend, Latinas as a group continue to have the highest rate of teen pregnancies overall (49.6 per 1,000) compared with Black (47.3 per 1,000), White (21.7), and Asian-Pacific groups (10.2, National Vital Statistics Report, 2013). Across Latin subgroups, Mexican-origin youth have the highest rate of pregnancy (73.0 per 1,000 ages 15–19), followed by Puerto Ricans (59.6) and Cubans (59.6, National Vital Statistics Report, 2013). Studies show higher rates of pregnancy for those residing in rural and urban neighborhoods, with segregation, lack of positive youth activities, and low family incomes correlated with higher rates of teen pregnancies (Center for Disease Control and Prevention, 2013).

Latino males report a higher rate of sexual risk taking than non-Latino Whites, with a greater likelihood of engaging in sexual intercourse without a condom (Centers for Disease Control and Prevention, 2007). Researchers have found that early involvement in sexual risk taking can be prognostic of continued problematic behaviors later in adolescent and adulthood (Windle, Mun, & Windle, 2005). Latina girls are particularly vulnerable to involvement with older men. Thirty-five percent of Latina youth reported engaging in sexual relations with a male four or more years her senior, compared to 11.9% non-Latina Black and 13.6% for non-Latina White youth (Abma, Martinez, Mosher, & Dawson, 2004). Research has shown that teens with partners who are four or five years their elder are more likely to engage in sexual activity, are less likely to use contraception, are more likely to get pregnant, are more likely to report later that they did not want to have sex that first time, and are likely to have more lifetime sexual partners (Albert, Brown, & Flanigan, 2003).

Such statistics present multiple issues for young Latinas. Early motherhood can pose multiple stressors, acting as both a cause and a consequence of poverty. It also prevents many young women from obtaining an education and participating in the work force. Finally, researchers have found that children born to teen mothers are at a higher risk for poverty themselves, and often experience greater health, behavioral, and educational problems later in life (Hoffman, 2006).

Racial/Ethnic Discrimination

Myriad studies have documented the discrimination experienced by Latino/as of all generations (Chithambo, Huey, & Cespedes-Knadle, 2014). Forms of discrimination can vary, from overt formations such as profiling/hassling by the police, exclusion or mistreatment by peers, teachers, and community members, and more severe sentencing in the legal system (Malott, 2010; Raby, 2012; The Sentencing Project, 2010). However, racism is also experienced by Latino/a youth in subtle formations, reflected in the attitudes and assumptions others have about a person simply due to his or her appearance. In a study of Latino/a strengths and challenges (Malott, 2010), one Mexican American adolescent described the many stereotypes directed toward her by the Whites in her community: "Just because you're Mexican [people assume] you're undocumented, taking away the jobs, you're one of those gangster people who steal, who get high . . . you're gonna drop out . . . you're gonna be pregnant" (p. 14). Such stereotypes, when held by educators, can lead to lowered academic and career expectations for Latino/a youth, whereby youth experience invisibility in the classroom, as teachers ignore them in spite of their raised hands (Malott, 2010).

Empirical evidence has shown unequal treatment, including dispro- portionally punitive punishment (Sáenz & Ponjuan, 2011) and tracking of Latino/a youth into lower-level, non-college courses across school systems (Samson & Lesaux, 2008). A recent national survey revealed that Latino/a parents were aware of this. When asked, Latino/a parents reported that their children were unfairly labeled learning disabled or incorrectly identified with behavioral problems. They also perceived that many teachers had lowered expectations of their children, or that many lacked the ability to work with children from different cultures (Pew Hispanic Center, 2004).

Such experiences have been described by many Latino/as, youth and adults, in our own studies in various locations across the country. For instance, in one study (Malott, 2010), multiple students discussed the phenomenon of lowered teacher and counselor expectations in their schools, including inap- propriate placement into lower-level or English-learning courses, or guidance toward what students perceived as lower-track courses and less prestigious post-secondary options. Some expressed frustration that they were behind aca- demically due to that discrimination. As one student who experienced place- ment into low-level courses explained, "In this school district, not many of my type made it very far, sadly . . . it took a while to get back on par, and I [still] don't think I'm on par" (p. 16). Another described his reaction to his counselor's suggestion that he attend a smaller, less prestigious college than his preferred choice, noting, "When I walked out [of the counselor's office] I was laughing, because I knew . . . she was going to tell me that, because it was something that they told my sister, also" (pp. 16–17).

Researchers have posited that a link exists between negative schooling experiences for youth of color and poor academic performance (Monroe, 2005), school dropout, and even delinquency (Monroe, 2005; Noguera, 2003; Voelkl, Welte, & Wieczorek, 1999). Discrimination has been linked to additional and multiple negative outcomes for Latino/a individuals. Examples include lower self-esteem (Moradi & Risco, 2006), psychological stress related to a sense of powerlessness, invisibility, and loss of integrity (Sue, Capodilupo, & Holder, 2008), reduced academic motivation, lower grade point averages, reduced academic well-being (Alfaro, Umaña-Taylor, Gonzales-Backen, &

Bámaca, 2009), depression, risky behaviors (Behnke, Plunkett, Sands, & Bámaca-Colbert, 2011; Delgado, Updegraff, Rosa, Umaña-Taylor, 2011), attention deficit hyperactivity disorder, conduct disorder, oppositional defiant disorder (Coker et al., 2009), panic disorder, substance use, anxiety, smoking, and suicide ideation (Ai, Aisenberg, Weiss, & Salazar, 2014; Chithambo et al., 2014; Lorenzo-Blanco & Cortina, 2013). Experts have noted subtle forms of racial and ethnic discrimination as equally harmful to individuals as more overt formations (Sue et al., 2008), with ongoing exposure to discrimination in its varying forms potentially effecting trauma-like symptomology (Goodman & West-Olatunji, 2010) and stress-related diseases (e.g., high blood pressure, hypertension, stroke, and cardiovascular disease; Blascovich, Spencer, Quinn, & Steele, 2001; Clark & Gochett, 2006; Merritt, Benett, Williams, Edwards, & Soller, 2006).

Nonetheless, Latino/a youth with adult support and encouragement have shown the ability to thrive in the face of discrimination (Harper & Associates, 2014). Youth of color have cited the desire to prove others wrong in overcoming negative group stereotyping (Malott, 2010). Researchers have also found that strong ethnic identities can act as a barrier to discrimination (Ai et al., 2014), and Latino/as with pride in their race or ethnicity are often shown to possess more active coping strategies to such stressors. Examples of active coping responses include thoughts or actions that counter harmful acts or statements (Phinney & Chavira, 1995; Umaña-Taylor, Vargas-Chanes, Garcia, & Gonzales-Backen, 2008).

In-Group Discrimination and Conflict

As has been noted before, there is great diversity among and across the various Latino/a subgroups. At times, and for varying reasons, these differences may lead to conflict. Examples include prejudices regarding perceived and real differences, and the desire to maintain pride in unique identities based on national origins (Portes & Rumbaut, 1996). There are also issues of hierarchy, whereby subgroups attempt to position themselves as 'better' than other Latino/a subgroups in an effort to obtain greater access to societal resources. An example of this is the prejudice related to skin color. Such a perspective, brought by many Latino/a immigrants from their home countries (Oboler, 1995), is highlighted in a dominant U.S. society that accords those with lighter skin tones with the greatest privileges. Hence, a hierarchy of racial preference is perpetuated across all racial groups in the United States, significantly impacting intragroup relations (Uhlmann, Dasgupta, Elgueta, Greenwald, & Swanson, 2002).

Conflicts between Latino/as of the same origins also exist. At times, this can be political. For instance, during one interview with a Mexican-origin youth (Malott, 2005), the young woman explained that she avoided one Latino peer due to his activist stance, exemplified in his chosen label of *Chicano*: "Sometimes, the Chicanos that I have met, they have so much pride in who they are, that they take that too far." Within-group conflicts can also fall along generational lines. In that same study, another young woman described her arrival in the U.S. and the conflict experienced with her same-origin peers:

> There were only two or three Hispanic kids with me in the whole school. But they were Mexican American. They had been here, you know, maybe [two] generations. So I . . . was from Mexico, therefore I was Mexican . . . I didn't understand the animosity that that would create among the people that had been here already. Because there's just so much stress between Hispanics, you know, second generation with first-generation Hispanics. They actually wanted to beat me up after school on my first day.

Familial Acculturation Clashes

Youth whose parents are foreign born face unique challenges. They are often expected to act as a bridge between parents and the host society, forcing them into an adult role as they translate language and culture to their caretakers (Quinones-Mayo & Dempsey, 2005). However, as youth begin to adopt U.S. norms, a process dubbed *acculturation*, they may begin to clash with their parents' traditional beliefs and expectations. Adolescents may be especially prone to high-risk behaviors due to this familial conflict (Le & Stockdale, 2008), potentially feeling misunderstood and isolated from familial support. That isolation is further exacerbated if language barriers exist between parent and child, limiting parent-child ability to connect, while deterring parents from reaching out for support from monolingual English-speaking teachers and counselors.

This phenomenon was powerfully illustrated in a focus group study of Latino/a immigrant mothers (Quinones-Mayo & Dempsey, 2005), whereby a tearful mother described the behaviors of her "Americanized" (p. 650) teenage girl. The girl rarely spoke to her mother, calling her "old fashioned" (p. 650). She lied about her whereabouts to spend time with friends. She shouted at her mother, insisting she "had a right to lead her own life" (p. 650). In one instance, the authors described supportive responses from the other Latina mothers in the focus group:

Each mother in turn acknowledged their feelings of emptiness and their pain of loss, each agreeing that the real problem was this country and, more so, social workers who (often in school) urged the children to express themselves and denigrate parental authority. And so begins the search for the bicultural balance between immigrant Latino/a families and their "American" adolescents.

(p. 650)

Youth with foreign-born parents may feel trapped between seemingly contradictory parental and societal norms. Whichever norms prevail, a potential challenge could emerge. For instance, traditional Latino/a norms regarding gender roles, promoted by family and Latino/a communities and peers, can at times negatively impact youth achievement. Expectations for boys and girls differ, with caretaking in the male role framed in terms of earning money to help support family (affiliated with the positive aspects of *machismo*). For both women and men, the Latino/a value of loyalty and staying close to, and caretaking, family may play into decisions such as high school dropout or the refusal to pursue a college degree. As described by one young man at a symposium on school dropout (The College Board Advocacy and Policy Center, 2010):

Machismo and familismo are major issues in Latino/a communities. Be a strong male . . . mask your emotions. And be loyal and responsible to the family. You're expected to work and contribute to the family—very much along the line of traditional gender roles and expectations.

(p. 11)

Foreign-Born Youth: Legal and Acculturation Challenges

Foreign-born youth possess a unique strength in that they often bring with them pride in, and a solid sense of, their culture and traditions. This includes a strong sense of connection to their families, which in turn provide support for those youth, acting as a buffer against environmental stressors (Boutakidis, Guerra, & Soriano, 2006). Hence, researchers have found that foreign-born youth have lower rates of at-risk behaviors, such as drug use, than their more acculturated or "Americanized" peers (Gfroerer & Tan, 2003). However, this group also experiences stressors unique to their generational status.

For instance, foreign-born youth may exhibit PTSD-like symptoms due to traumatic migration experiences, resulting in poorer levels of physical and psychological health (Torres & Wallace, 2013). If migrating alone or with one or two family members, they will often lack support in their new setting (Williams, 2003), in turn leaving them more vulnerable to exploitation and abuse by the adults around them (Dirks-Bihun, 2014). Foreign-born youth experience higher rates of stress related to acculturation, whereby they must learn to adapt to a new culture. This may, at times, leave them feeling marginalized, and societal negative attitudes toward immigrants may compound that sense of isolation. That risk is particularly exacerbated for those who lack English language skills, as many do, with approximately 70% of this population indicating that they speak English less than "very well" (U.S. Census Bureau, 2011).

Living in the U.S. with an undocumented status impacts both the mental and emotional health of Latino/a youth (Gonzales, Suárez-Orozco, & Dedios-Sanguineti, 2013). Sources of distress include: impaired freedom or mobility due to the inability to legally work and, in some states, obtain a driver's license; discrimination (Flores et al., 2008); low social status (Alegria et al., 2007); higher rates of poverty due to undocumented status (U.S. Census Bureau, 2004b); and limited access to health, educational, and social resources (Mirowsky & Ross, 2003; Phelan, Link, & Tehranifar, 2010). Additionally, undocumented families have less access to public programs, and youth often face school disruption or financial hardship, should parents lose their jobs due to immigration enforcement and/or deportation (The Annie E. Casey Foundation, 2014). The constant threat of deportation, either of themselves or their loved ones, forces youth to experience continuous feelings of fear, stress, and anxiety (Bernal et al., 2010).

Educational attainment is a challenge for foreign-born Latino/as. Approximately one out of two (52%) foreign-born Latino/as never complete high school, compared to 25% of those who are native born (Pew Hispanic Center, 2010). Factors that lead to school dropout have been cited as schooling difficulties before migration, racial and ethnic biases, and poverty and the ensuing need to work (Pew Hispanic Center, 2005). Language has also been shown as a factor in school completion; one statistic indicated that 15% of Latino/as aged 16–19 who were fluent in English did not graduate from high school, while more than 59% of Latino/a English language learners of the same age group had dropped out (Fry, 2003).

Latino/a immigrants who do persist in school may experience many challenges, including lower skills based on poor school experiences in their home country, culturally and linguistically biased testing, lowered academic expectations of teachers, and the inability of teachers to bridge the cultural divide between themselves and foreign-born students (Pew Hispanic Center, 2004). Students may also experience acculturative stress related to an attempt to balance loyalty to familial culture, language, and traditions with pressures to conform to differing peer, school, and work expectations (Holleran & Waller, 2003; Rumbaut, 2005).

Each year, approximately 650,000 undocumented immigrants graduate high school only to face barriers to advancement in their education which, in turn, offers little to no options for climbing out of poverty (Abrego & Gonzales, 2010). Activists have proposed the Development, Relief, and Education for Alien Minors legislative proposal (better known as the DREAM act), yet to be approved, as a means of allowing citizenship for undocumented youth. The Deferred Action for Childhood Arrivals (DACA) policy was recently approved by the U.S. government, granting undocumented youth the right to apply for temporary work permits, although without granting legal status to a person (Immigration Policy Center, 2013). Hence, for current, undocumented youth who do go on to college, they must fund their own schooling, and they cannot be legally employed in the U.S. upon earning a degree. Funding one's own schooling often requires working long hours, leaving youth disconnected from peers and campus resources and support (Bernal et al., 2010). In interviews with undocumented Latino/as attending college (Bernal et al., 2010), one youth, named Patricio, described the struggles he faced:

> A challenge that I face, of course, is financial aid, with not qualifying for money, and work-study is involved. I mean I would have so much free time to do activities with a job on campus. Since I don't have that, I have to go to Spokane every day and work. Then by the time I get out of work, the school offices are closed and my professors are gone. I never have the time to go to a club meeting or just wander around campus [and] talk to people.
>
> (pp. 620–621)

CHALLENGES: RESPONSE AND TOOLS

Researchers have identified the many stressors and barriers facing Latino/a youth in their environments, including school, community, and home settings. Children of color across many groups, including African American youth, are also disproportionately impacted by many of the same barriers (e.g., discrimination, segregation, and poverty). Hence, a logical and ideal solution is for all to work together to remove the many barriers that prevent so many of our youth from achieving their career and educational goals. Such effort may entail challenging discriminatory educational policies and cultural norms, and altering laws, policies, and practices that sustain segregation and poverty across entire neighborhoods and their affiliated schools. We must all work to redress the many inequalities that affect our nation's children and, by default, the future economic stability and growth of the nation itself (The Education Trust, 2013).

However, within the scope of this book, some of the greatest work we can do is to build up our youth and their identities, to offer resiliencies and tools for survival and success in society. We must understand that internal and contextual strengths already exist, to remember that individuals of Latino/a descent are already succeeding against the odds with the assistance of strong communities and families (Telzer, Gonzales, & Fuligni, 2014). Our job is to tap into those many resources and strengths, largely found in familial cultural values, norms, and traditions, to further encourage that success. This is not the complete answer to the many challenges faced by this population, but it is an important one. Hence, the group sessions in this book are designed with the intent to draw from cultural strengths, to inform youth lifestyles and decision making.

REFERENCES

Abma, J. C., Martinez, G. M., Mosher, W. D., & Dawson, B. S. (2004). *Teenagers in the United States: Sexual activity, contraceptive use, and childbearing, 2002*. National Center for Health Statistics. Vital Health Statistics 23(24). Retrieved from http://www.cdc.gov/nchs/data/series/sr_23/sr23_024.pdf

Abrego, L. J., & Gonzales, R. G. (2010). Blocked paths, uncertain futures: The postsecondary education and labor market prospects of undocumented Latino/a youth. *Journal of Education for Students Placed at Risk, 15*, 144–157. doi:10.1080/10824661003635168

Ai, A. L., Aisenberg, E., Weiss, S. I., & Salazar, D. (2014). Racial/ethnic identity and subjective physical and mental health of Latino/a Americans: An asset within? *American Journal of Community Psychology, 53*, 173–184. doi:10.1007/s10464-014-9635-5

Albert, B., Brown, S., & Flanigan, C. (Eds.) (2003). *14 and younger: The sexual behavior of young adolescents*. Washington, DC: National Campaign to Prevent Teen Pregnancy.

Alegria, M., et al. (2004). Considering context, place and culture: The National Latino/a and Asian American Study. *International Journal of Methods in Psychiatric Research, 13*(4), 208–220.

Alfaro, E. C., Umaña-Taylor, A. J., Gonzales-Backen, M. A., Bámaca, M. Y., & Zeiders, K. H. (2009). Latino/a adolescents' academic success: The role of discrimination, academic motivation, and gender. *Journal of Adolescence, 32*, 941–962. doi:10.1016/j.adolescence.2008.08.007

The Annie E. Casey Foundation. (2014). *Race for results: Building a path to opportunity for all children*. Retrieved from www.kidscount.org

Baum, S., & Flores, S.M. (2011). Higher education and children in immigrant families. *Future Child, 21*(1), 171–193. Retrieved from http://futureofchildren.org/publications/journals/article/index.xml?journalid=74&articleid=545

Behnke, A. O., Plunkett, S. W., Sands, T., & Bámaca-Colbert, M. Y. (2011). The relationship between Latino/a adolescents' perceptions of discrimination, neighborhood risk, and parenting on self-esteem and depressive symptoms. *Journal of Cross-Cultural Psychology, 42*, 1179–1197. doi:10.1177/0022022110383424

Bernal, D. D., Alemán, E., & Garavito, A. (2010). Latina/o undergraduate students mentoring Latina/o elementary students: A borderlands analysis of shifting identities and first-year experiences. *Harvard Educational Review, 79*, 560–585. Retrieved from http://www.hepg.org/her-home/home

Blascovich, J., Spencer, S. J., Quinn, D., & Steele, C. (2001). African Americans and high blood pressure: The role of stereotype threat. *Psychological Science, 12*, 225–229. doi:10.1111/1467-9280.00340

Bloom, S. L. (2005). Creating sanctuary for kids: Helping children to heal from violence. *Therapeutic Community: The International Journal for Therapeutic and Supportive Organizations, 26*(1), 57–63. Retrieved from http://www.sanctuaryweb.com/PDFs_new/Bloom%20Intro%20Creating%20Sanctuary%20for%20Children%20TC.pdf

Boutakidis, I., Guerra, N. G., & Soriano, F. (2006). Youth violence, immigration, and acculturation. In N. G. Guerra & E. P. Smith (Eds.), *Preventing youth violence in a multicultural society* (pp. 75–100). Washington, DC: American Psychological Association.

Bryan, J., Moore-Thomas, C., Day-Vines, N. L., & Holcomb-McCoy, C. (2011). School counselors as social capital: The effects of high school college counseling on college application rates. *Journal of Counseling & Development, 89*(2), 190–199. doi:10.1002/j.1556-6678.2011.tb00077.x

Caughy, M., O'Campo, P., & Muntaner, C. (2003, July). When being alone might be better: Neighborhood poverty, social capital, and child mental health. *Social Science & Medicine, 57*, 227–237. doi:10.1016/S0277-9536(02)00342-8

Center for Disease Control and Prevention. (2013). *CDC features: Teen birth rates drop, but disparities persist.* Retrieved from http://www.cdc.gov/features/dsTeenPregnancy/

Chithambo, T. P., Huey, S. J., & Cespedes-Knadle, Y. (2014). Perceived discrimination and Latino/a youth adjustment: Examining the role of relinquished control and sociocultural influences. *Journal of Latina/o Psychology, 2*, 54–66. doi:10.1037/lat0000012

Clark, R., & Gochett, P. (2006). Interactive effects of perceived racism and coping responses predict a school-based assessment of blood pressure in Black youth. *Annals of Behavioral Medicine, 32*, 1–9. doi:10.1207/s15324796abm3201_1

The College Board Advocacy and Policy Center (2010). The educational crisis facing young Men of Color. Retrieved from www.collegeboard.com/advocacy

Coker, T. R., Elliott, M. N., Kanouse, D. E., Grunbaum, J. A., Schwebel, D. C., Gilliland, M. J., et al. (2009). Perceived racial/ethnic discrimination among fifth-grade students and its association with mental health. *American Journal of Public Health, 99*, 878–884. doi:10.2105/AJPH.2008.144329

Darling-Hammond, L. (2004). What happens to a dream deferred? The continuing quest for educational equality. N. J. A. Banks & C. M. Banks (Eds.), *Handbook of research on multicultural education* (2nd ed., pp. 607–632). San Francisco, CA: Jossey Bass.

Davis, T. M., & Welcher, A. N. (2013). School quality and the vulnerability of the black middle class: The continuing significance of race as a predictor of disparate schooling environments. *Sociological Perspectives, 56*(4), 467–493. doi:10.1525/sop.2013.56.4.467

Delgado, M. Y., Updegraff, K. A., Roosa, M. W., & Umaña-Taylor, A. J. (2011). Discrimination and Mexican-origin adolescents' adjustment: The moderating roles of adolescents', mothers', and fathers' cultural orientations and values. *Journal of Youth and Adolescence, 40*, 125–139. doi:10.1007/s10964-009-9467-z

Dirks-Bihun, A. (March/April 2014). Immigration and sexual abuse: Protecting undocumented children. *Social Work Today*, 22–25. Retrieved from www.socialworktoday.com

Eaton, S. R. (2011). *How long does it take to learn a second language? Applying the "10,000-hour rule" as a model for fluency.* Retrieved from http://www.eric.ed.gov/PDFS/ED516761.pdf

The Education Trust. (2013). *Breaking the glass ceiling of achievement for low-income students and students of color.* Retrieved from https://www.txcharterschools.org/files/media/BreakingtheGlassCeiling_052013-20130516-100546.pdf

Flores, E., Tschann, J. M., Dimas, J. M., Bachen, E. A., Pasch, L. A., & de Groat, C. L. (2008). Perceived discrimination, perceived stress, and mental and physical health among Mexican-Origin adults. *Hispanic Journal of Behavioral Sciences, 30*(4), 401–424. doi:10.1177/0739986308323056

Fry, R. (2003). *Hispanic youth dropping out of U.S. schools: Measuring the challenge.* Washington, DC: Pew Hispanic Center. Retrieved from http://pewhispanic.org/files/reports/19.pdf

Fry, R., & Taylor, P. (2013). Hispanic high school graduates pass Whites in rate of college enrollment. Retrieved from http://www.pewhispanic.org/2013/05/09/hispanic-high-school-graduates-pass-whites-in-rate-of-college-enrollment/

Gfroerer, J. C., & Tan, L. L. (2003). Substance use among foreign-born youths in the United States: Does the length of residence matter? *American Journal of Public Health, 93*(11), 1892–1895. Retrieved from http://ajph.aphapublications.org/

Gonzalez, J. (August 2010). *Reports highlight disparities in graduation rates among White and minority students.* Retrieved from Chronicle of Higher Education website: http://chronicle.com/article/Reports-Highlight-Disparities/123857/

Gonzales, R. G., Suárez-Orozco, C., & Dedios-Sanguineti, M. C. (2013). No place to belong: Contextualizing concepts of mental health among undocumented immigrant youth in the United States. *American Behavioral Scientist, 57*(8), 1174–1199. doi:10.1177/0002764213487349

Goodman, R. D., & West-Olatunji, C. A. (2010). Educational hegemony, traumatic stress, and African American and Latino/a American students. *Journal of Multicultural Counseling and Development, 38*, 176–186. doi:10.1002/j.2161-1912.2010.tb00125.x

Greenstone, M., & Looney, A. (2013). *Thirteen economic facts about social mobility and the role of education.* Retrieved from the Hamilton Project website http://www.hamiltonproject.org/papers/thirteen_economic_facts_social_mobility_education/

Harper, S. R., & Associates (2014). *Succeeding in the city: A report from the New York City Black and Latino/a male high school achievement study.* Retrieved from http://www.gse.upenn.edu/equity/nycreport

Harvard Graduate School of Education (2011). *Pathways to prosperity.* Retrieved from http://www.gse.harvard.edu/news_events/features/2011/Pathways_to_Prosperity_Feb2011.pdf

Hoffman, S. (2006). *By the numbers: The public costs of teen childbearing.* Retrieved from campaign@teenpregnacy.org

Holleran, L. K., & Waller, M. A. (2003). Sources of resilience among Chicano/a youth: Forging identities in the borderlands. *Child and Adolescent Social Work Journal, 20*, 335–350. doi:10.1023/A:1026043828866

Hopper, E. K., Bassuk, E. L., & Olivet, J. (2010). Shelter from the storm: Trauma-Informed Care in homelessness services settings. *The Open Health Services and Policy Journal, 3*, 80-100. Retrieved from http://www.benthamscience.com/open/tohspj/

Hoxby, C. H., & Turner, S. J. (2013). *Informing students about their college options: A proposal for broadening the expanding college opportunities project.* Retrieved from http://www.hamiltonproject.org/files/downloads_and_links/THP_ HoxbyTurner_FINAL.pdf

Immigration Policy Center (2013). How DACA is impacting the lives of those who are not DACAmented: Preliminary findings from the National UnDACAmented Research Project. Retrieved from http://www.immigra tionpolicy.org/sites/default/files/docs/daca_final_ipc_csii_1.pdf

Jacobson, R. (March 2014). Should children take antipsychotic drugs? *Scientific American, 25*(2). Retrieved from http://www.scientificamerican. com/article/should-children-take-antipsychotic-drugs/

Le, T. N., Stockdale, G. (2008). Acculturative dissonance, ethnic identity, and youth violence. *Cultural Diversity and Ethnic Minority Psychology, 14*, 1–9. doi:10.1037/1099-9809.14.1.1

Lorenzo-Blanco, E. I., & Cortina, L. M. (2013). Towards an integrated under- standing of Latino/a/a acculturation, depression, and smoking: A gendered analysis. *Journal of Latina/o Psychology, 1*, 3–20. doi:10.1037/a0030951

Phelan, J. C., Link, B. G., & Tehranifar, P. (2010). Social conditions as fundamental causes of health inequalities: Theory, evidence, and pol- icy implications. *Journal of Health and Social Behavior, 51*, S28–S40. doi:10.1177/0022146510383498

Malott, K. (2005). Ethnic self-labeling in the Latina population (Doctoral dissertation, University of Northern Colorado, 2005). *Dissertation Abstracts International*, 66, 1284.

Malott, K. M. (2010). Being Mexican: Strengths and challenges of Mexican- origin adolescents. *Journal of School Counseling, 8*(12). Retrieved from http:// jsc.montana.edu/

Merritt, M. M., Benett, G. G., Williams, R. B., Edwards, C. L., & Soller, J. J. (2006). Perceived racism and cardiovascular reactivity and recovery to personally relevant stress. *Health Psychology, 25*, 364–369. doi:10.1037/ 0278-6133.25.3.364

Mirowsky, J., & Ross, C. E. (Ed.) (2003). *Social Causes of Psychological Distress* (2nd ed.). New York, NY: Walter de Gruyter, Inc.

Monroe, C. R. (2005). Why are the "bad boys" always Black? Causes of dis- proportionality in school discipline and recommendations for change. *The Clearing House, 79*, 45–50. Retrieved from https://www.theclearinghouse.org/

Moradi, B., & Risco, C. (2006). Perceived discrimination experiences and mental health Latino/a/a American persons. *Journal of Counseling Psychology, 53*, 411–421. doi:10.1037/0022-0167.53.4.411

Moreno, C. (2012). Hispanic education and employment: Aligning college degrees with workforce needs. *The Huffington Post*. Retrieved from http:// www.huffingtonpost.com/

National Center for Education Statistics (2013). *Digest of Education Statistics 2012*. Washington, DC: U.S. Department of Education. Retrieved from http://nces.ed.gov/programs/digest/

National Commission on Teaching and America's Future (January 2003). *No dream denied: A pledge to America's children*. Washington, DC: National Committee on Teaching and America's Future. Retrieved from http://nctaf.org/wp-content/uploads/2012/01/no-dream-denied_summary_report.pdf

National Vital Statistics Report (2013). *Births: Final data for 2011* (Volume 2, Number 61). Retrieved from http://citeseerx.ist.psu.edu/viewdoc/download?doi=10.1.1.309.1435&rep=rep1&type=pdf

Noguera, P. A. (2003). Schools, prisons, and social implications of punishment: Rethinking disciplinary practices. *Theory Into Practice, 42*, 341–350. doi:10.1207/s15430421tip4204_12

Oboler, S. (1995). *Ethnic labels, Latino/a lives: Identity and the politics of (re)presentation in the United States*. Minneapolis, MN: University of Minnesota Press.

Ozer et al. (2011). Does delivering preventive services in primary care reduce adolescent risky behavior? *Journal of Adolescent Health, 49*, 476–482. doi:10.1016/j.jadohealth.2011.02.011

Pew Hispanic Center (2004). *National Survey of Latino/as: Education*. Washington, DC: Pew Hispanic Centre. Retrieved from http://pewhispanic.org/files/reports/25.pdf

Pew Hispanic Center (2005). *Hispanics: A people in motion*. Retrieved from http://pewhispanic.org/files/reports/40.pdf

Pew Hispanic Center (2010). *Hispanics, high school dropouts and the GED*. Retrieved from http://www.pewhispanic.org/2010/05/13/hispanics-high-school-dropouts-and-the-ged/

Pew Hispanic Center (2012). *Hispanic student enrollments reach new highs in 2011*. Retrieved from http://www.pewhispanic.org/2012/08/20/hispanic-student-enrollments-reach-new-highs-in-2011/

Phinney, J. S., & Chavira, V. (1995). Parental ethnic socialization and adolescent coping with problems related to ethnicity. *Journal of Research on Adolescence, 5*, 31–53. doi:10.1207/s15327795jra0501_2

Policy Link (2011). *California's tomorrow: Equity is the superior growth model*. Policy Link and USC Program for Environmental and Regional Equity. Retrieved from http://www.policylink.org/site/c.lkIXLbMNJrE/b.7843037/k.1048/Americas_Tomorrow_Equity_is_the_Superior_Growth_Model.htm

Portes, A., & Rumbaut, R. G. (1996). *Immigrant America: A portrait*. Berkeley, CA: University of California Press.

Quinones-Mayo, Y., & Dempsey, P. (2005). Finding the bicultural balance: Immigrant Latino/a mothers raising "American" adolescents. *Child Welfare, 84*(5), 649–668. Retrieved from https://www.childwelfare.gov/

Raby, R. (2012). *School rules: Obedience, discipline and elusive democracy.* Toronto, Canada: University of Toronto Press.

Sáenz, V. B., & Ponjuan, L. (2011). *Ensuring the academic success of Latino/a males in higher education.* Washington, DC: Institute for Higher Education Policy. Retrieved from http://www.ihep.org/assets/files/publications/m-r/ (Brief)_Men_of_Color_Latino/as.pdf

Samson, J. F., & Lesaux, N. K. (2008). Language-minority learners in special education: Rates and predicators of identification for services. *Journal of Learning Disabilities, 48*(2), 148–162. doi:10.1177/002221940 8326221

Sapolsky, R. (December 2005). Sick of poverty. *Scientific American, 293,* 92–99. Retrieved from http://www.scientificamerican.com/

Sue, D. W., Capodilupo, C. M., & Holder, A. M. B. (2008). Racial microaggressions in the life experience of Black Americans. *Professional Psychology: Research and Practice, 39,* 329–336. doi:10.1037/0735-7028.39.3.329

Telzer, E. H., Gonzales, N., & Fuligni, A. J. (2014). Family obligation values and family assistance behaviors: Protective and risk factors for Mexican–American adolescents' substance use. *Journal of Youth and Adolescence, 43,* 270–283. doi:10.1007/s10964-013-9941-5

The Sentencing Project (2010). *Disproportionate minority contact.* Retrieved from http://www.ojjdp.gov/dmc/index.html

Therrien, M., & Ramirez, R. R. (2000). *The Hispanic Population in the United States: March 2000 (Current Population Reports,* pp. 250–535). Washington, D.C.: U.S. Census Bureau. Retrieved from http://www.census.gov/ prod/2001pubs/p20-535.pdf

Torres, J. M., & Wallace, S. P. (2013). Migration circumstances, psychological distress, and self-rated physical health for Latino/a immigrants in the United States. *American Journal of Public Health, 103*(9), 1619–1627. doi:10.2105/AJPH.2012.301195

Tuck, E. (2012). *Urban youth and school pushout: Gateways, get-aways, and the GED.* New York, NY: Routledge.

Uhlmann, E., Dasgupta, N., Elgueta, A., Greenwald, A. G., & Swanson, J. (2002). Subgroup prejudice based on skin color among Hispanics in the United States and Latin America. *Social Cognition, 20*(3), 198–225. doi:10.1521/soco.20.3.198.21104

Umaña-Taylor, A. J., Vargas-Chanes, D., Garcia, C. D., & Gonzales-Backen, M. (2008). A longitudinal examination of Latino/a adolescents' ethnic identity, coping with discrimination, and self-esteem. *Journal of Early Adolescence, 28*, 16–50. doi:10.1177/0272431607308666

U.S. Census Bureau (2004b). *The foreign-born population in the United States.* Retrieved from http://www.census.gov/prod/2004pubs /p20-551.pdf

U.S. Census Bureau (2011). *Language spoken at home: 2011 American community survey 1-year estimates.* Retrieved from http://www.census.gov/hhes/socdemo/language/data/acs/

U.S. Department of Education (2012). *New Americans in post-secondary education: A profile of immigrant and second-generation Americans.* Retrieved from nces.ed.gov

Vega, W. A., & Gil, A. G (1999). A model for explaining drug use behavior among Hispanic adolescents. *Drugs and Society, 14*, 47–74. doi:10.1300/J023v14n01_05

Voelkl, K. E., Welte, J. W., & Wieczorek, W. F. (1999). Schooling and delinquency among white and African American adolescents. *Urban Education, 34*, 69–88. doi:10.1177/0042085999341005

Williams, F. C. (2003). Concerns of newly arrived immigrant students: Implications for school counselors. *Professional School Counseling, 7*, 9–14. Retrieved from http://www.schoolcounselor.org/school-counselors-members/publications/professional-school-counseling-journal

Windle, E. Y., Mun, M., & Windle, R. C. (2005). Adolescent-to-young adulthood heavy drinking trajectories and their prospective predictors. *Journal of Studies on Alcohol, 66*, 313–322.

3

ETHNIC IDENTITY AND RESILIENCIES

Krista M. Malott and Tina R. Paone

*you don't really know
what you are. If you are
more mexican than american, sometimes
i think i am more mexican but
when i am in my social studies
class i begin to think how
am i Mexican? when i am learning
about american culture, and me not
knowing a thing about mexican
culture you don't really know
what you are when you are part
of two cultures*

Mexican-origin youth, Eastern Pennsylvania, 2009

Central to the core task of adolescent development is the achievement of both individual and social identities (Erikson, 1968; Tajfel, 1974). While dominant Western norms emphasize the development of the individual self, with individual-identity achievement related to the separation of self from the group, more collectivistic cultures (e.g., African, Asian, and Latin American) emphasize the collective "we" as most meaningful in informing one's identity and corresponding behaviors and well-being (Brewer & Chen, 2007). Ethnic identity is an essential aspect of social identity, entailing a sense of attachment and belonging to a particular ethnic group with a common ancestry (Phinney, 1989; Yip & Fuligni, 2002).

Shared traits across ethnic groups can include culture, values and customs, politics, history, religion, language, kinship, or place of origin (Phinney, 1996). Examples of ethnic groups include those according to country of origin (French Canadians, Dutch, Mexican, or Anglo Americans) or religion (e.g., Jewish, Amish; Giordano & McGoldrick, 1996). Ethnic identity is developed over time and through exploration. Exploration can include reading, talking to others, attending cultural events, or learning cultural practices, thereby increasing a person's knowledge regarding their group and leading to an increased (and conscientious) affiliation with and commitment to that group. One can be said to have achieved a strong sense of ethnicity if they identify strongly with that ethnic group following a period of identity exploration. Persons with strong ethnic identities will likely exhibit the following traits or behaviors (Phinney & Ong, 2007):

- Use of an ethnic label with personalized meaning (e.g., Latina, Hispanic, Pocho, Tica, etc.). It should be noted that label choices are diverse and dynamic across individuals, and some persons with strong ethnicities may even choose, for personal or political reasons, to eschew a label entirely. For those who assume a personal label, meanings and preferences for certain labels can differ across persons, time, and according to social situations (Malott, 2009).
- Participation in same-group behaviors or traditions. A person may possess a strong ethnic identity without engaging in same-group behaviors. However, persons with strong identities often seek connection with same-group members through shared activities or behaviors. Behaviors might include use of the group's language, eating group-specific foods, socializing with group members, and participating in group traditions.
- Shared values and beliefs. Values and beliefs can indicate a person's closeness to a group. This may include shared sociopolitical values, such as the belief that all Latino/a youth should have equal access to college funding, regardless of their immigration status. However, because ethnic groups are not monolithic in nature, values and beliefs can vary widely across individuals, and are particularly influenced by generational and immigration status, national origins, and socioeconomic status.

THE PROCESS OF ETHNIC IDENTITY DEVELOPMENT

Adolescence to young adulthood has been found to be a salient period for identity exploration. This may be particularly true in regards to the development of one's ethnic identity, as the pre-teen to young adult years entail increased exposure to different ethnic and racial groups through school changes and engagement in a wider range of academic and social activities. In turn, researchers have found that exposure to persons who are ethnically and racially different from oneself can prompt personal identity reflection (French, Seidman, Allen, & Aber, 2006).

Although Whites who are not of Latino/a descent also possess an ethnicity, ethnic identity tends to be a more salient factor for Latino/a youth (Rodriguez, Schwartz, & Whitbourne, 2010). This may be due to the discrimination experienced by those youth, which further serves to prompt self-reflection and exploration regarding ethnic group affiliation (Fuligni, Witkow, & Garcia, 2005). To illustrate, as one young Latina adolescent from a study (Malott, 2010) stated, "seeing that other people don't accept you . . . it just made me think more and more about [being Mexican] and eventually just to be even prouder" (p. 20). Pride in one's group can act as a protective agent for Latino/a youth against stressors such as discrimination, while providing a sense of belonging and acceptance that all individuals require in achieving a positive sense of well-being.

Following are the stages of ethnic identity development, according to expert Jean Phinney (1989), with comments from Latino/a youth who describe their own experiences of development at each stage:

1. **Unexamined ethnic identity.** The individual has not explored his or her ethnicity at this stage. The person may lack interest in discussing or thinking about this, with use of an ethnic label that has been assigned to them by external entities (e.g., the government, or parents). In this stage, if the person does affiliate with a group, it is without conscientious decision, usually because their family affiliates with the group.

   Fifteen-year-old Mexican American Ari (personal communication, 2005) represents an individual who is in this initial stage. When asked to respond to the question, "What does being Mexican mean to you?" there was a long pause, followed by the response; "I haven't thought about that . . . I have no idea." Lyda, age 34, reflecting on being in that initial stage of ethnic identity development in her high school years, explained, "When I was younger I used to say that I was . . . Chicana, and Latina, because I really didn't understand . . . what the terminology was and I didn't know how to identify myself. I really hadn't figured it all out yet."

2. **Ethnic identity search or moratorium.** At this stage, the individual may begin exploration of his or her identity, including exploration of

what it means to belong to one's ethnic group. Ethnic identity exploration is usually prompted by some event, such as exposure to different ethnic groups, discrimination from others outside of the group, or even same-peer prompting. Exploration may include reading, talking to others, thinking about the meaning of one's identity in context, learning cultural practices, and attending cultural events.

As an example of an individual at this stage, Juan, a participant in a 2009 interview (personal communication), described initiating his exploratory period with friends at age 12, beginning with discussions regarding ethnic labels and their meanings: "Me and my friends . . . we used to think about . . . what we wanted to be, and one of my friends just asked, what we consider ourselves?" In another interview (personal communication, 2005), Alicia, 19, described the sources that influenced her ethnic identity development during her exploratory period in late high school and early college:

> I took this class and we learned a lot about where people in Mexico came from, and all Southern American countries. And then, just some people that I know that I talk to and the way they see themselves and why they do that. Just learning, from even reading a text book.

3. **Ethnic identity achievement.** At this stage, the individual has searched and achieved a clear, positive, and confident sense of his or her ethnicity, with an understanding and knowledge regarding one's group traits/ practices. The person usually experiences a pride in, and commitment to, one's heritage, with a sense of belonging to a specific group. A poignant comment by 14-year-old Mexican American Gina, in an interview with Malott (personal communication, 2006), illustrates an achieved status:

> I took the time to research my heritage, to find out who I was, to find out where I came from and who my people were. Somebody who does do that I think should be really proud of themselves.

It should be noted that individuals may not always develop a strong or positive sense of ethnicity, particularly if they internalized a negative sense of their own group (e.g., internalized discrimination). To illustrate this, in one study (Malott, 2006), a Latina woman in her sixties described early, traumatic experiences of discrimination toward herself and her same-ethnic peers at school: "[We] got smacked around if they spoke Spanish. [We] were sent home . . . beaten up . . . spit on" (p. 86). As a result of those experiences, she internalized a negative sense of her ethnicity and had yet to advance beyond the first level of ethnic identity development. Conversely, another participant in her early thirties in the same study noted that, upon having children, she experienced a surfacing of pride and a desire to better understand and engage in her ethnic group traditions, so that she might pass on such pride and practices to her own children. Hence, ethnic identity development is a unique process, influenced by individual and contextual factors, and ever-changing across one's lifespan.

RESEARCH AND ETHNICITY

Ethnic identity has been shown to impact a vast array of factors in the lives of Latino/a youth. For instance, a strong and positive ethnic identity has been shown to act as a buffer to stressors or to societal problems (Kiang, Yip, Gonzales-Backen, Witkow, & Fuligni, 2006; Mossakowski, 2003; Phinney & Rotheram, 1987; Quintana, 2007). It has been correlated with self-rated mental and physical health (Ai et al., 2014), wellness (Rayle & Myers, 2004), sense of well-being (Smith & Silva, 2011; Umaña-Taylor, 2004; Yip & Fuligni, 2002), a high quality of life (Utsey, Chae, Brown, & Kelly, 2002), and higher self-esteem (Bracey, Bámaca, & Umaña-Taylor, 2004; Phinney & Alipuria, 1990; Phinney, Cantu, & Kurtz, 1997). Those with stronger ethnic identities have shown a lowered risk of drug use (Belgrave, Townsend, Cherry, & Cunningham, 1997), improved coping strategies (McMahon & Watts, 2002), and greater academic achievement and social success (Ong, Phinney, & Dennis, 2006).

As a result of such findings, professor and scholar Holcomb-McCoy (2005) asserted that the "failure of an adolescent to examine ethnic issues and his or her ethnic identity creates risks for poor psychological and education adjustment" (p. 124). In turn, it has been suggested that counselors should emphasize the ethnic identity development of youth of color in helping them face a multitude of barriers experienced in society. A group setting has been suggested as a meaningful forum for addressing the topic of ethnic identity (Baca & Koss-Chioino, 1997; Rivera, 2004) which, in turn, inspired the creation of this very book.

ETHNICITY VERSUS RACE

People, scholars included, have a tendency to confuse the constructs of race and ethnicity. Although there is overlap in those identities, it is important to understand that they are distinct from one another (Smedley & Smedley, 2005). Race, largely recognized as a socially constructed phenomenon, rather than one that is inherently biological, is generally used to refer to one's skin tone. Ethnicity encompasses a group of persons with similar traditions, values, or beliefs who may differ from one another racially (Helms, 2002; Neville, Worthingnton, & Spanierman, 2001). Hence, a Latino who identifies with a Panamanian ethnicity may have dark skin and therefore consider himself racially Black. Conversely, a lighter-skinned peer who is also of Panamanian origin may racially self-identify as White.

Part of the confusion and controversy over the meaning of race and ethnicity stems from history. Who has been allowed to self-ascribe racially as White, and therefore receive the many privileges associated with Whiteness, has varied over the history of the United States. For instance, in the early history of the nation, many Eastern European immigrants were not considered part of the White race, and certain laws defining Whiteness have varied widely across individual states, so that person's assigned race changed as they crossed state lines (Campbell, 2009). Today, race as a construct remains highly contested, largely due to the recognition of the privileges still accorded to those with lighter skin tones (Jones, 2013). While the U.S. Census recognizes the term Latino/a as denoting an ethnic group, others have argued for and against categorizing Latino/as under the racial category of Whiteness (Yancey, 2003). What is certain is that Latino/as can experience discrimination related to their ethnicity and racism related to their skin color.

Discussions concerning race and ethnicity can be lively and informative for young Latino/as during group sessions. Such conversations can acknowledge and explore conflicting opinions, as well as encourage the development of uniquely chosen racial and ethnic labels that represent a pride in self and identity (e.g., such as *Blaxican*, indicating a Black and Mexican heritage). Ultimately, being proud of one's self racially *and* ethnically can provide protective barriers against the many stressors experienced by adolescents of tone (Brook & Pahl, 2005).

PRO-LATINO/A: IS IT ANTI-AMERICAN?

Empirical evidence presented in this book hopefully demonstrates that youth can benefit from knowing, and being proud of, their ethnic heritage. However, this may contradict what many of us have been told regarding success in the U.S. Upon arriving in the U.S., immigrants and their children have received implicit (and sometimes very explicit) messages that social and material success is achieved through forsaking knowledge and pride in one's immigrant roots, and instead embracing the dominant language, culture, history, and heritage (a viewpoint called *assimilation*). This belief in assimilation was powerful enough to inspire passage of an Arizona bill in 2012 (Planas, 2013) that made it illegal in that state to offer any kind of educational experience specific for ethnic groups, on the grounds that such material could "promote the overthrow of the U.S. government, [and] foster racial resentment" (para. 5).

However, as researchers have come to show, a strong ethnic identity can provide a much-needed tool of support and defense against the many stressors experienced by Latino/a youth. In addition, the argument that strengthening one's ethnic identity will promote hatred or resentment toward others is counter to what we know about identity development. According to racial identity development theories, as individuals become positive and strong in their own identities, their perceptions of other racial groups can positively improve (Atkinson, Morten, & Sue, 1998). In our own ethnic identity group study (Malott, Paone, Humphreys, & Martinez, 2010), we found that as Latino/a youth learned more about their own ethnic group, their opinions toward Whites were positively impacted. Representative statements reflecting this included:

- [Through group participation, I] learned not to discriminate against Whites.
- [I learned in group] not to be so racist, to not dislike the gringos [e.g., Whites].
- [I learned in group] to get along better with them [Whites] (p. 262).

Hence, such findings suggest that a strong ethnic identity, whereby youth value and know their heritage, improves relationships with both self and others. The ideal identity status entails embracing one's own heritage *in addition* to selectively incorporating dominant heritage beliefs and practices, as a kind of *bicultural* status (Berry, 1997). Research has shown that such selective biculturalism allows Latino/as to live healthier lifestyles, often because they are able to choose the most beneficial practices from two cultures (Lagana, 2003). Latino/a youth in many of our studies noted that a bicultural status could be beneficial. This even has positive career implications, as Christie, a young Latina (Malott, personal communication, 2005), explained:

> For me, Chicana is not one-hundred percent Mexican, it's not one-hundred per-cent American . . . Which gives me a perfect future, 'cause I know English and Spanish, which will give me . . . a really good college degree and everything, which would help me out, and being Chicana helps me translate for other peo-ple, understand people, and talk back to people.

Finally, it is important to acknowledge the challenges associated with being in that middle space, whereby at times a youth may feel distant from those who solely identify with dominant (e.g., U.S.) or Latino/a norms (Berry, 1997). Biculturalism, when experienced as 'in the middle,' can be a lonely place, and isolation can negatively impact one's mental and physi-cal health. Christie goes on to explain this: "It is hard being in the mid-dle . . . first because you don't get the full American experience and you don't get the full Mexican experience. You are in the middle and taking a little bit of both, you cannot take them all and sometimes it's . . . hard to deal with" (personal communication, 2005). Ideally, professionals can help youth experiencing this sense of marginalization to identify and explore this struggle, as well as to connect with similar others—those who are also in 'the middle.'

COUNSELOR ETHNIC IDENTITY

Over the years, in implementing counseling groups and research interviews with Latino/a youth regarding ethnic identity topics, it hasn't been uncom-mon for those youth to turn a wary eye our way, to respond with questions such as: "What ethnic label do *you* use?" "What's *your* immigration history?" "What do *you* know about racism?" or "What values are important to *you*?" They had an excellent point—why should they self-disclose personal or potentially sensitive information that we, ourselves, were unwilling to share as group facilitators? Particularly because, as adults and as Whites, we had the power in those situations.

Indeed, written and verbal feedback from several youth who participated in our ethnic identity groups showed that the facilitator's self-disclosure regarding topics such as racism and White privilege, immigrant history, and personal ethnicity was considered meaningful to them. Group facilita-tors also perceived that their own participation in certain activities, whereby they briefly presented some facet and meaning of their ethnic identities, was received by the adolescents with great interest. In turn, the adolescents responded with an equal level of depth and seriousness in discussing their own selves. Hence, group facilitators were able to model knowledge and meaning that was then mirrored in the youths' responses.

To be able to model such knowledge and meaning, a group facilitator would of course need to possess a developing, if not strong, ethnic identity. To increase personal knowledge of topics such as ethnic labeling, discrimination, and immigration history, facilitators will likely need to engage in an exploratory process. That may include returning to the source (e.g., immigration history) of one's arrival of family members to the U.S. Following is a set of questions we encourage group facilitators to explore, through journaling or discussion, to better know one's self and, in turn, better facilitate youth in learning about themselves.

- Consider the stages of ethnic identity development (Phinney, 1989), briefly described below and in greater detail earlier in the chapter. What stage are you at?

  - Unexamined ethnic identity. At this stage, the individual has little to no exploration of his or her ethnicity.
  - Ethnic identity search or moratorium. The individual begins a personal search regarding his or her identity (usually prompted by an event, such as this book).
  - Ethnic identity achievement. The individual has explored and achieved a clear, positive, and confident sense of his/her ethnicity.

- At what age did you begin to become aware of your ethnic identity?

  - Who or what prompted this awareness?

- What are your origins (e.g., your immigration history)?

  - When did your ancestors arrive in the U.S., and why did they immigrate?
  - What was their immigrant experience like (getting here)?
  - When they arrived, did they experience persecution, prejudice? Preferential treatment?
  - How does any of the above impact you now?

- Which languages did your family speak?

  - Do they still speak them, or are there phrases or expressions that your family continues to use?

- What values and traditions does your family honor?

  - Which are related to your immigrant origins?
  - How do they shape your behaviors and identity?

- What biases may you have inherited from family regarding other ethnic groups?

  - How might that impact your work with persons from those groups?

- What religion(s) have ancestral family members practiced?

  - How does religion inform your life now?

- What else has been passed down through your family that may be related to your immigrant roots (e.g., hobbies, foods, stories, knowledge, histories, and tragedies)?

  - How have these made you who you are today?

- What is your current ethnic label?

  - What does your label mean to you? To others in your family?
  - Who inspired you to use this label?
  - If you do not have a label, what meaning do you make of that?

- How have others viewed your ethnic group, presently and historically?

  - How has society's treatment of your group affected you or your family?
  - How can the historical discrimination against your own immigrant group inform your understanding of discrimination experienced by Latino/a youth today?

- How do you feel about belonging to your own ethnic group(s)?

  - Do you share this information with others, and if so, who and when?
  - Do you hide it from some others, and if so, when and why?

- What *race* do you consider yourself?

  - What is your racial label, and what does it mean?
  - What racial category do others put you in, and how does it make you feel?
  - What race was your family considered, historically, when people from your group first began immigrating to the United States (this may require research)?
  - How does your race connect with your ethnicity, if at all?
  - How do you have racial privilege, or lack of? How does this impact your life?
  - How do you cope with racial privilege or oppression personally experienced?
  - What biased perceptions might you have learned regarding other racial groups?

- If you were unable to answer any of these questions, talk or journal about how that feels.

  ❏ What has kept you from learning this information about yourself?
  ❏ To whom can you go for certain answers, or to which resources can you refer?
  ❏ If you are unable to recover your history, discuss what this means to you. What has replaced that history, culture, knowledge?

Exploration of such questions is a large undertaking, and one that, if done well, could take a lifetime. In group work that draws on clients' ethnic identities to explore life choices and behaviors, that self-knowledge is essential for group facilitators. At times, facilitators may need to model sharing of personal knowledge with brief self-disclosure. At other times, knowledge about one's self will serve to increase a facilitator's comfort level in guiding identity-related discussions with group members. No matter one's age or education level, openness to additional professional and personal exploration of the topic can benefit helpers both personally and professionally.

REFERENCES

Ai, A. L., Aisenberg, E., Weiss, S. I., & Salazar, D. (2014). Racial/ethnic identity and subjective physical and mental health of Latino/a Americans: An asset within? *American Journal of Community Psychology, 53*, 173–184. doi:10.1007/s10464-014-9635-5

Atkinson, D. R., Morten, G. M., & Sue, D. W. (1998). *Counseling American minorities: A cross cultural perspective* (5th ed.). Dubuque, IA: Brown: William C. Brown Publishers.

Baca, L. M., & Koss-Chioino, J. D. (1997). Development of a culturally responsive group counseling model for Mexican American adolescents. *Journal of Multicultural Counseling and Development, 24*, 130–141. doi:10.1002/j.2161-1912.1997.tb00323.x

Belgrave, F. Z., Townsend, T. G., Cherry, V. R., & Cunningham, D. M. (1997). The influence of an Africentric worldview and demographic variables on drug knowledge, attitudes, and use among African American youth. *Journal of Community Psychology, 25*, 421–433. doi:10.1002/(SICI)1520-6629(199709)25:5

Berry, J. W. (1997). Immigration, acculturation, and adaptation. *Applied psychology: An International Review, 46*(1), 5–33. doi:10.1111/j.1464-0597.1997.tb01087.x

Bracey, J. R., Bamaca, M. Y., & Umaña-Taylor, A. J. (2004). Examining ethnic identity and self-esteem among biracial and monoracial adolescents. *Journal of Youth and Adolescence, 33,* 123–132. doi:10.1023/B:JOYO. 0000013424.93635.68

Brewer, M., & Chen, Y. (2007). Where (who) are collectives in collectivism? Toward conceptual clarification of individualism and collectivism. *Psychological Review, 114,* 133–151. Retrieved from http://www.apa.org/pubs/journals/rev/

Brook, J. S., & Pahl, K. (2005). The protective role of ethnic and racial identity and aspects of an Africentric orientation against drug use among African American young adults. *The Journal of Genetic Psychology, 166*(3), 329–345. doi:10.1097/PSY.0b013e3182583a50

Campbell, G. R. (2009). Many Americas: The intersection of class, race, and ethnic identity. In A. L. Ferber, C. M. Jiménez, A. O'Reilly Herrera, & D. R. Samuels (eds.), *Examining the dynamics of oppression and privilege* (pp. 198–225). Boston, MA: McGraw Hill.

Erikson, E. H. (1968). *Identity: Youth and crisis.* New York, NY: Norton.

French, S. E., Seidman, E., Allen, L., & Aber, L. J. (2006). The development of ethnic identity during adolescence. *Developmental Psychology, 42,* 1–10. doi:10.1037/0012-1649.42.1.1

Fuligni, A. J., Witkow, M., & Garcia, C. (2005). Ethnic identity and the academic adjustment of adolescents from Mexican, Chinese, and European backgrounds. *Developmental Psychology, 41,* 799–811. doi:10.1037/0012-1649.41.5.799

Giordano, J., & McGoldrick, M. (1996). European families: An overview. In M. McGoldrick, J. Giordano, & J. K. Pearce (eds.), *Ethnicity and family therapy* (pp. 427–441). New York, NY: Guilford.

Helms, J. E. (2002). A remedy for the Black-White score disparity. *American Psychologist, 57,* 303–305. Retrieved from http://www.ncbi.nlm.nih.gov/pubmed/11975388

Holcomb-McCoy, C. (2005). Ethnic identity development in early adolescence: Implications and recommendations for middle school counselors. *Professional School Counseling, 9,* 120–127.

Jones, J. (2013). *A dreadful deceit: The myth of race form the colonial era to Obama's America.* New York, NY: Basic Books.

Kiang, L., Yip, T., Gonzales, M., Witkow, M., & Fuligni, A. (2006). Ethnic identity and daily psychological well-being of adolescents from Mexican and Chinese backgrounds. *Child Development, 77,* 1338–1350. doi:0009-3920/2006/7705-0016

Lagana, K. (2003). Come bien, camina, y no se preocupe—eat right, walk and do not worry: Selective biculturalism during pregnancy in a Mexican

American community. *Journal of Transcultural Nursing, 14*, 117–124. doi:10.1177/1043659602250629

Malott, K. (2005). Ethnic self-labeling in the Latina population (Doctoral dissertation, University of Northern Colorado, 2005). *Dissertation Abstracts International, 66*, 1284.

Malott, K. M. (2009). Investigation of ethnic self-labeling in the Latina population: Implications for counselors and counselor educators. *Journal of Counseling & Development, 87*, 179–185. doi:10.1002/j.1556-6678.2009. tb00565.x

Malott, K. M. (2010). Being Mexican: Strengths and challenges of Mexican-origin adolescents. *Journal of School Counseling, 8*(12). Retrieved from http://jsc.montana.edu/

Malott, K. M., Paone, T. R., Humphreys, K., & Martinez, T. (2010). Use of group counseling to address ethnic identity development: Application with adolescents of Mexican descent. *Professional School Counseling, 13*(5), 257–267. Retrieved from http://www.schoolcounselor.org/school-counselors-members/publications/professional-school-counseling-journal

McMahon, S. D., & Watts, R. J. (2002). Ethnic identity in urban African American youth: Exploring links with self-worth, aggression, and other psychosocial variables. *Journal of Community Psychology, 30*, 411–431. doi:10.1002/jcop.10013

Mossakowski, K. N. (2003). Coping with perceived discrimination: Does ethnic identity protect mental health? *Journal of Health and Social Behavior, 44*, 318–331. Retrieved from http://www.jstor.org/stable/1519782? origin=JSTOR-pdf&

Neville, H. A., Worthingnton, R. L., & Spanierman, L. B. (2001). Race, power, and multicultural counseling psychology: Understanding White privilege and color-blind racial attitudes. In J. P. Ponterotto, J. M. Casas, L. A. Suzuki, & C. M. Alexander (eds.), *Handbook of multicultural counseling* (2nd ed., pp. 257–288). Thousand Oaks, CA: Sage.

Ong, A., Phinney, J., & Dennis, J. (2006). Competence under challenge: Exploring the protective influences of parental support and ethnic identity in Latino/a college students. *Journal of Adolescence, 29*, 961–979. doi:10.1016/j.adolescence.2006.04.010

Phinney, J. S. (1989). Stages of ethnic identity development in minority group adolescents. *Journal of Early Adolescence, 9*, 34–49. doi:10.1177/0272431689091004

Phinney, J. S. (1996). When we talk about American ethnic groups, what do we mean? *American Psychologist, 51*, 918–927. doi:0003-066X/96/$2.00

Phinney, J. S., & Alipuria, L. L. (1990). Ethnic identity in college students from four ethnic groups. *Journal of Adolescence, 13*, 171–183. doi:10.1016/0140-1971(90)90006-S

Phinney, J. S., & Ong, A. D. (2007). Conceptualization and measurement of ethnic identity: Current status and future directions. *Journal of Counseling Psychology, 54*(3), 271–281. doi:10.1037/0022-0167.54.3.271

Phinney, J. S., Rotheram, M. J. (eds.). (1987). *Children's ethnic socialization: Pluralism and development*. Newbury Park, CA: Sage.

Phinney, J. S., Cantu, C. L., & Kurtz, D. A. (1997). Ethnic and American identity as predictors of self-esteem among African Americans, Latino/a, and White adolescents. *Journal of Youth and Adolescence, 26*, 165–183. Retrieved from http://www.springer.com/psychology/child+%26+school+psychology/journal/10964

Planas, R. (March, 2013). Arizona's law banning Mexican-American studies curriculum is constitutional, judge rules. *Huffington Post*.

Quintana, S. M. (2007). Racial and ethnic identity: Developmental perspectives in research. *Journal of Counseling Psychology, 54*, 259–270. doi:10.1037/0022-0167.54.3.259

Rayle, A. D., & Myers, J. E. (2004). Counseling adolescents toward wellness: The roles of ethnic identity, acculturation, and mattering. *Professional School Counseling, 8*, 81–91. Retrieved from http://www.schoolcounselor.org/school-counselors-members/publications/professional-school-counseling-journal

Rivera, E. T. (2004). Psychoeducational and counseling groups with Latino/as. In C. R. Kalodner, M. T. Riva, J. L. DeLucia-Waak, & D. A. Gerrity (eds.), *Handbook of group counseling and psychotherapy* (pp. 213–223). Thousand Oaks, CA: Sage.

Rodriguez, L., Schwartz, S. J., & Whitbourne, S. K. (2010). American identity revisited: The relation between national, ethnic, and personal identity in a multiethnic sampling of emerging adults. *Journal of Adolescent Research, 25*(2), 324–349. doi:10.1177/0743558409359055

Smedley, A., & Smedley, B. D. (2005). Race as biology is fiction, race as a social problem is real: Anthropological and historical perspective on the social construction of race. *American Psychologist, 60*, 16–26. doi:10.1037/0003-066X.60.1.16

Smith, T. B., & Silva, L. (2011). Ethnic identity and personal well-being of people of color: A meta-analysis. *Journal of Counseling Psychology, 58*(1), 42–60. doi: 10.1037/a0021528

Tajfel, H. (1974). Social identity and intergroup behavior. *Social Science Information, 13*, 65–93. doi:10.1177/053901847401300204

Umaña-Taylor, A. J. (2004). Ethnic identity and self-esteem: Examining the role of social context. *Journal of Adolescence, 27*, 139–146. doi:10.1016/j.adolescence.2003.11.006

Utsey, S. O., Chae, M. H., Brown, C. F., & Kelly, D. (2002). Effects of ethnic group membership on ethnic identity, race-related stress and quality of life. *Cultural Diversity & Ethnic Minority Psychology, 8*, 366–377.

Yancey, G. (2003). *Who is White? Latino/as, Asians and the new Black/Non-Black divide.* Boulder, CO: Lynne Reiner Publishers Inc.

Yip, T., & Fuligni, A. J. (2002). Daily variation in ethnic identity, ethnic behaviors, and psychological well-being among American adolescents of Chinese descent. *Child Development, 73*, 1557–1572. doi:0009-3920/2002/7305-0016

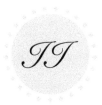

GROUP SESSIONS

The following chapters provide a set of experiential group sessions, each addressing different topics. The first set is focused on facilitating youth exploration of their ethnic identities, while connecting this identity with myriad tenets such as career and life goals and tactics in confronting and coping with discrimination. This chapter is premised on the literature that supports ethnic identity as a key underlying construct in Latino/a youth success, and for that reason, this is the first set of sessions in the book.

Subsequent chapters continue to draw from Latino-specific cultural practices and issues while addressing distinct areas, from healthy relationships, to grief, to the strengthening of youth agency. As noted earlier in the book, some sessions may work better when used together, as a series of sessions that build upon one another (such as the Hope group sessions in Chapter 7). At other times, sessions can be pulled out and adapted for a single event.

Many of the chapters include handouts for the youth, to define topics or illustrate concepts, and are bilingual. It should be noted that many of the sessions have been successfully applied with boys and girls of various ages (from 8 to 18). The key is to adapt content to youth-specific traits, from language, cultural values and traditions, and contextual stressors, to youth strengths and developmental levels.

LATINO/A YOUTH AND ETHNIC IDENTITY DEVELOPMENT

Krista M. Malott and Tina R. Paone

SESSION 1: WHERE ARE YOU GOING AND HOW WILL YOU GET THERE?

Part of this session is adapted from Butterfly Beginnings, Jones 1998

Session Goal: To identify and share personal life goals and barriers to goal achievement.

Time Needed: 30–45 minutes

Suggested Group Size: 2–15

Materials Needed:

- Brown paper lunch bags
- Writing utensils
- Markers/colored pencils/crayons
- Piece of paper for each member with the outline of a butterfly on it
- Two ropes or strings to create river banks. For youth ages 6–10, create the river banks approximately 12 feet wide—wider for older youth, to offer a greater challenge to them
- Three short pieces of wood or cardboard
- Blank paper

Session Directions:

- Give each group member a brown paper lunch bag and instruct them to write their name on the outside of the bag.
- Butterfly outlines should be given to each member. Ask each to write a specific and realistic life goal inside or near the butterfly, giving examples (e.g., to be more patient; graduate; improve at math; argue less with mom).
- Direct them to decorate their butterflies. When completed, have them place them inside their bags.
- Indicate that the bag represents a cocoon, explaining what a cocoon is.
- Seal up bags, and place them on the other side of the 'river bank' constructed with rope.
- Ask group members to stand on one side of the river, across from their cocoons/goals, and announce: "We're on one side of a river bank and the river is full of angry alligators. On the other side is the person we want to become and the goals we want to achieve. The goal is crossing as a team without touching as much as a toe into the water. If one person touches the water, she/he is eaten by the alligator and you all have to return to start over. It takes the help of others to become the best we can become, so you're going to work as a team. Feel free to be as creative as you want."
- During the activity, the group facilitator should write members' statements on a piece of paper ("Oh!" "Shoot!" "That was dumb" "What a great idea," etc.).
- If you see members touch the water, ask the whole group to start the process over.
- After all members have crossed the river, process the experience with the questions below.
- After processing, ask members to open their bags and read their goals to one another. Urge them to hang goals up at home, to inspire them.

Process Questions:

1. What was required from the group for everyone to get to the other side?
   ¿Qué se requirió del grupo para que todos cruzaran al otro lado del río?

2. Good teams are supportive. Does it sound like you were supportive in your comments to one another? (read back comments you recorded)
   En un buen equipo los miembros se apoyan el uno al otro. ¿Te parece que ustedes se apoyaron en los comentarios que se dieron?

3. In real life, we need help to cross our own personal river of alligators to get to our goals. Who keeps you strong and helps you do that?
    En la vida real, necesitamos ayuda para cruzar nuestro propio río de caimanes para alcanzar nuestras metas. ¿Quién te mantiene fuerte y te ayuda en ese camino?

4. Who is on your team that might actually keep you from reaching your goal?
    ¿Quién en tu grupo puede evitar que alcances tus metas?

5. Achieving a goal takes small steps. What is your first step?
    Alcanzar una meta requiere varios pasos. ¿Cuál sería tu primer paso?

6. This activity said you were 'crossing a river of alligators.' In real life, who or what are the challenges that might slow you down in reaching your goals?
    En esta actividad se dijo que estabas 'cruzando un río de caimans.' En la vida real, quiénes o cuáles son los desafíos que pueden interferir al alcance de tus metas?

7. Are there barriers related to being Latino/a that might create an obstacle to reaching your goal?
    ¿Hay obstáculos relacionados al ser Latino/a que pueden crear una barrera al alcance de tus metas?

8. What strengths regarding being Latino/a will help you overcome barriers and reach your goal?
    ¿Cuáles ventajas en ser Latino/a te ayudarán a superar estos obstáculos y alcanzar tus metas?

SESSION 2: CALL ME THIS, CALL ME THAT

Session Goal: To strengthen group members' knowledge related to ethnicity.

Time Needed: 40–50 minutes

Suggested Group Size: 2–15

Materials Needed:

- Index cards
- Writing utensils
- Playing cards (Appendix A)
- Label clarifications/definitions (Appendix B)
- Masking or heavy tape
- Black/whiteboard or paper

Session Directions:

- Ask members to shout out all the ethnic labels they have heard to represent their group, without exploring label meanings. Write each on an index card as you hear it called out.
- Tape one of the cards to each member's backs, without them seeing which it is.
- Ask them to look at one another's labels and silently consider the meanings of each.
- Explain that you will play a game, during which they should treat others according to that group member's assigned label placed on their back.
- Instruct members to choose a playing card (Appendix A) from the pile, read directions out loud, and follow the directions.
- At the end of the game, have each person try to guess the label on his/her back, asking them to explain how they came to that conclusion.
- Have them define all the labels' meanings (opinions will likely differ).
- Provide additional label clarifications/definitions, referring to Appendix B.

Process Questions:

1. What feelings do you have about how you were treated because of your label?
   ¿Cómo te sientes sobre la forma que has sido tratado(a) por la manera que te han catalogado?

2. What label do you feel other people have given you?
   ¿Cómo crees que otras personas te han catalogado?

3. Who do you label in real life?
    ¿A quién le pones una etiqueta étnica en la vida real?

4. Why do we put labels on others and how do you feel about this?
    ¿Por que catalogamos a otras personas y cómo te sientes sobre ello?

5. Labels can be good, too . . . when can they be good?
    ¿La manera en que catalogamos a las personas también puede ser positiva . . . en que situación lo puede ser?

6. What labels were you given as a Latino/a, specifically (if any)?
    ¿Cómo te han catalogado específicamente por ser Latino/a?

7. What will your label be, if you choose to use one? Why?
    ¿Cómo te catalogarías, si tuvieras que escoger una etiqueta? ¿Por qué?

8. What's most important to you about what we talked about today?
    ¿Qué es lo más importante para ti de lo que hemos hablado en el día de hoy?

SESSION 3: THE VALUES TREE

Session Goal: To identify and explore meaningful cultural values.

Time Needed: 40–55 minutes

Suggested Group Size: 2–15

Materials Needed:

- Large construction paper
- Scissors
- Tape/glue
- Craft materials, as desired (glitter, feathers, macaroni, pipe cleaners, etc.)
- Index cards
- Markers/colored pencils/crayons
- A board or poster board with examples and definitions of values (Appendix C)

Session Directions:

- Divide into smaller groups (maximum three per group).
- Explain that each small group will create a 'values tree.'
- Direct members to use construction paper and craft materials to create the basic outline of a very large tree of any shape, about half as tall as they are, with large roots at the bottom.
- Once they have completed their trees, introduce the concept of values, asking for, and offering, specific examples and definitions (see Appendix C).
- Review the definitions of gender roles (machismo/marianismo, Appendix C) and discuss their views of those definitions.
- Ask group members to shout out all the values that seem important to them, family members, or peers. Write them on a board as they brainstorm out loud. This may include: values they learned growing up; *dichos* (proverbs) they learned; values regarding how men and women behave.
- Hand each group member two blank index cards and ask them to write their most important dichos and/or values on their cards.
- Once group members have completed these value cards, have them glue/tape them at the roots of their tree.
- Ask members to write in the leaves or branches how their 'root' values helped their 'tree grow,' and give an example (e.g., if someone put in their roots the dicho 'work before play,' perhaps in a branch they would

write as an outcome of this value 'hard worker,' 'good group member,' or 'get good grades').

■ Once the trees have been completed, have the smaller groups present and explain their creations.

Process Questions:

1. From whom did you learn your values?
   ¿De quién aprendiste tus valores?

2. Which values are most important to you? Why?
   ¿Cuáles son los valores más importantes para ti? ¿Por qué?

3. Which value or values do you wish you could follow better?
   ¿Cuáles valores deserías seguir mejor?

4. What keeps you from following certain value(s)?
   ¿Qué no te permite seguir ciertos valores?

5. Tell us about values that others noted today that you would like to possess or that you found interesting.
   ¿Qué nos puedes decir sobre los valores que otros señalaron hoy los cuales te gustaría poseer, o que te parecieron interesantes?

6. What are your beliefs regarding how Latino/as should behave, including their roles in the family?
   ¿Cuáles son tus creencias sobre como se deben comportar los Latino/as, incluyendo sus funciones en la familia?

7. From whom did you learn this?
   ¿De quién has aprendido esto?

8. What are your thoughts/feelings about these expected gender roles or behaviors?
   ¿Qué piensas sobre el papel o comportamiento previsto para cada género?

Facilitator Notes: Find a way to preserve or display the values trees, perhaps asking the youth what they would like to do with them.

SESSION 4: LATINO/A HEROES

Session Goal: Identify positive role models and determine how they inspire achievement.

Time Needed: 10–15 minutes

Suggested Group Size: 2–15

Materials Needed:

- Photos of historical or contemporary Latino/a figures (selected to match the group's ethnic origins), with 2–3 inspirational facts about each of them
- Scissors
- Construction paper
- Tape/glue
- Paint
- Markers/colored pencils/crayons
- Craft materials, as desired (glitter, feathers, macaroni, pipe cleaners, etc.)

Session Directions:

- Ask group members to shout out names of Latino/as who have made history or inspired others. Invite them to consider people in their families, communities, and schools. Share the Latino/a role models you have.
- Write the names on a board or paper for all to see, exploring how those persons act as positive role models (see process questions below).
- Ask them to each create a mask, using the available crafts, making representations of their role model(s) or what they have learned, or gained, from that role model(s).
- Allow ample time for the creation, encourage creativity, and stress that they do not have to create a mask that looks exactly like the role model(s).
- After the masks are complete, allow each group member to share and explain his/hers.

Process Questions:

1. What do you think makes someone a role model?
   ¿En tu opinión que hace que una persona sea un modelo a seguir?

2. What are the qualities of a role model?
   ¿Cuáles son las cualidades de un un modelo a seguir?

3. Are your role models positive? Negative? How so? What have they taught you?

   ¿Cómo son tus modelos a seguir? ¿Son positivos o negativos? Explica. ¿Qué te han enseñado ellos?

4. Have any of these role models faced tough times? How did they deal with them?

   ¿Estos modelos a seguir han tenido que enfrentar momentos difíciles? ¿Cómo le hicieron frente?

5. In what way might your role model inspire you to be better?

   ¿En que manera te puede inspirar un modelo a seguir para que seas mejor?

6. Who are your role models that have taught you what it means to be Latino/a?

   ¿Quiénes son los modelos a seguir que te han enseñado el significado de ser Latino/a?

7. How are you a role model to others?

   ¿Cómo eres tú un modelo a seguir para otras personas?

8. What might you do, to become a better role model?

   ¿Qué harías para convertirte en un mejor modelo a seguir?

Facilitator Notes: Encourage group members to display their masks at home, to inspire them to overcome and achieve in tough times.

SESSION 5: WRITE IT OR RAP IT

Session Goal: To creatively express Latino/a identities and experiences.

Time Needed: 40–50 minutes

Suggested Group Size: 2–15

Materials Needed:

- Two to three age-appropriate poems about Latino/a identity, such as those from the book, *Red Hot Salsa: Bilingual Poems on Being Young and Latino in the United States* (Carlson, 2005). One copy of each poem for each member
- Blank paper
- Writing utensils
- Board/large notepad
- Copies of song lyrics and a song recording (if possible) that addresses identity or experience of Latino/as in the U.S. (such as *Mohado,* by Ricardo Arjona)

Session Directions:

- Ask group members to read a poem and explore its possible meanings and the emotion it evokes.
- Have members read the lyrics to a selected song while the recording is playing.
- Ask group members to talk about what the lyrics mean to them.
- Ask them to name other artists who relate their life struggles powerfully.
- In dyads or alone, ask members to write their own story, rap, or song, with a focus on their identities or experiences as Latino/as.
- Have members read or perform their work to the larger group.
- Discuss some of the powerful messages or feelings that emerged.

Process Questions:

1. Was it difficult or easy to think about what makes you special as a Latino/a?
   ¿Fue fácil o difícil pensar en lo que te hace especial por ser Latino o Latina?

2. Why did you choose the words you did?
   ¿Por qué escogiste esas palabras para describirte?

3. Was anyone surprised by any of the poems or songs?
   ¿Se sorprendió alguien sobre algunos de los poemas o canciones?

4. What did you like that you heard others talk about?
   ¿Qué te gustó sobre las conversaciones que oiste?

5. What was hard to hear or write about?
   ¿Qué te fue difícil oír o escribir?

6. Do you think being Latino/a is different for males and females, and did that come out in your poems, songs, or raps? How so?
   Piensas que ser Latino/a es diferente para las mujeres y los hombres, ¿Cómo se manifestó esto en tus poemas o canciones?

SESSION 6: STANDING UP TO THE BAD

Adapted from The Good, the Bad, & the Ugly, Jones 1998

Session Goal: To learn new ways to respond to negative peer influences and life barriers.

Time Needed: 40–50 minutes

Suggested Group Size: 2–15

Materials Needed:

- Blank paper, index size, approximately eight pieces per youth
- Writing utensils
- A box or bag labeled 'good'
- A box or bag labeled 'bad'
- Scenarios (examples in Appendix D) written in English and Spanish

Session Directions:

- Explain that you will practice good and bad ways to deal with barriers.
- Ask group members to define and give examples of barriers experienced in life (if they cannot, provide some: things, events, or persons that can make life harder for us or keep us from getting what we want. Examples might include racism, living in poverty, or bullies).
- Pass out eight pieces of paper to each member, to allow for four good and four bad solutions.
- Explain that they will be given a scenario that presents a barrier (see Appendix D for examples, or tailor your own to the population). Have group members take turns reading a scenario in both English and Spanish, and after each one, ask them to write one good and one bad solution to each on separate pieces of paper (give examples for the first one). Then ask them to place them in the appropriately labeled box.
- Ask one of the group members to pull out one card from the bad box and read a solution. Discuss why it might be a 'bad' solution. Review a good solution next.
- When completed, ask group members to pick what they feel was the best solution.
- Have them practice (role play) the best solution in dyads or as a whole group.
- Move to a second scenario and repeat the process as desired.

Process Questions (after each scenario):

1. How was this activity?
   ¿Cómo fue esta actividad para ti?

2. What most stood out to you?
   ¿Qué fue lo que se destacó más para ti?

3. Was it easy or hard to do it the 'good' way? Why?
   ¿Fue fácil o difícil hacerlo de la manera 'correcta'? ¿Por qué?

4. Would you normally do it that way? If not, why not?
   ¿Usualmente lo harías de esa manera? ¿Por que sí o por qué no?

5. Do you think you will use this good way in real life?
   ¿Piensas que vas a usar esta "manera buena" en la vida real?

6. How do you know something is a good solution versus a bad solution?
   ¿Cómo distingues entre una buena solución y una mala solución?

7. What do you want to use that we talked about today, when it comes to barriers?
   ¿Qué te gustaría hacer sobre lo que hemos hablado hoy en lo que se refiere a enfrentando barreras?

REFERENCES

Carlson, L. M. (Eds.) (2005). *Red hot salsa: Bilingual poems on being young and Latino in the United States.* New York, NY: Henry Holt and Company.

Jones, A. (1998). *The wRECking yard.* Ravensdale, WA: Idyll Arbor, Inc.

TABLE 4.1 LABEL PLAYING CARDS

Shake the hand of the person whose label you most appreciate or like. Do not use their label, but explain why you like this label best.	*Dale la mano a la persona que tiene la "etiqueta" que tú aprecias más. No uses la etiqueta pero explica porque te parece la mejor.*
Choose the person with the label that you feel would most make people angry or upset. Without saying what the label is, explain why the label might make some people angry/upset. Do you agree and feel the same?	*Escoge la persona que tiene la "etiqueta" que tú crees le molestaría a muchas personas. Sin decir cuál es la etiqueta explica porqué esta clasificación le molestaría a algunas personas. ¿Estás tú de acuerdo o te sientes de la misma manera?*
Pick one person whose label is new for you, or you have no idea what it means. Ask others to define it, without using the label.	*Escoge a una persona cuya etiqueta es nueva para ti, o no tienes ni idea de lo que significa. Pídele a otros que la definan, sin necesidad de utilizar la etiqueta.*
Announce: Everybody stand up and give a high-five to one person who you feel is most similar to you, according to labels. Then explain to the group why you high-fived that person, without using their label.	*Anuncia: Todos levántense y denle la mano a una persona que creen se asemeja más a ustedes de acuerdo a su clasificación. Luego explícale al grupo porque le diste la mano a esa persona sin usar su etiqueta.*
Sit next to the person you think is most different from you, based on their label. Explain why you chose this person, but do not use his or her label.	*Siéntate al lado de la persona que tú crees ser más diferente a ti basado en como la han catalogado. Explica porque escogiste a esta persona, pero no uses la etiqueta que le han dado.*
Pick who your *mother or father* would most want you to be friends with, in the group, according to that person's label. Without using the label, explain why your parents would prefer a person who is labeled that way.	*Escoge a alguien del grupo a quien tu madre o a tu padre le gustaría que fueras su amigo/a de acuerdo a como le han catalogado. Sin mencionar la etiqueta, explica porque tus padres preferirían una persona que sea catalogada así.*
Choose two people who you think would be closest friends, according to their labels. Ask them to shake hands. Without using their labels, explain why you chose them.	*Escoge a dos personas las cuales crees serían mejores amigos de acuerdo a su etiqueta. Pídeles que se den la mano. Sin usar la etiqueta que les han dado, explica porque las escogiste.*
Pick a person who you believe is *very* Latino/a, according to his or her label, and ask him/her to stand while you explain why you consider him/her *very* Latino/a.	*Escoge a una persona quien tú crees es muy Latino/a de acuerdo a su etiqueta y pídele que se levante mientras les explica el porque lo/la consideras 'muy' Latino/a.*

Definitions of Labels

- **Latino/a:** 1. American Spanish, probably short for Latino/a Americano (Latin American). Other definitions: a native or inhabitant of Latin America. 2. a person of Latin American origin living in the U.S. 3. a person of Cuban, Mexican, Puerto Rican, South or Central American, or other Spanish culture of origin, regardless of race.
  Latino/a: 1. Latinoamericano/a. Otras definiciones: un nativo o habitante de Latinoamérica. 2. Una persona de origen Latinoamericano que vive en los Estados Unidos. 3. Una persona de origen cubano, mexicano, puertorriqueño, sur o centroamericano, o de otra cultura de origen español sin importar la raza.

- **Hispanic:** A term selected by a group of governmental experts (Latino/as and non-Latino/as), refers to all Spanish-speaking communities from across Latin America. Latino/as tend to reject the government-imposed term.
  Hispano: Una palabra seleccionada por un grupo de expertos gubernamentales (de Latinos y no Latinos), que se refiere a todas las comunidades hispano hablantes de toda Latinoamérica. Los Latino/as suelen rechazar esta palabra impuesta por el gobierno.

- **Chicano:** Generally used to describe a person of Mexican descent born in the U.S. Chicana and Chicano became popular during the *Chicano political movement* of the 1960s and 1970s as Mexican Americans tried to find a cultural and political identity for themselves.
  Chicano: Una palabra generalmente usada para describir a una persona de origen mexicano nacida en los Estados Unidos. Las palabras chicano y chicana se hicieron populares durante el movimiento político chicano de los años sesenta y setenta cuando los mexicoestadounidenses trataban de encontrar una identidad cultural y política.

Example Dichos *(Proverbs) and Values and Gender Roles*

Examples of *dichos* (proverbs):

- *Cuando una puerta se cierra, otra se abre* (When one door closes, another one opens)
  [value: optimism, good can come from the bad]
- *No se le puede pedir peras al olmo* (You cannot ask an elm tree to bear pears)
  [value: pragmatism/practicality, we should have realistic expectations]
- *A la mejor cocinera se le escapa un tomate* (Even the best cook can lose a tomato)
  [value: compassion, we all make mistakes]

Examples of values frequently identified by Latino/a individuals:

- *Familismo* (importance of family and extended kinship relationships)
- *Respeto* (respect)
- *Machismo* (traditional male role)
- *Solidaridad* (being united with and supportive of your group)
- *Marianismo* (traditional female role)
- *Dignidad* (treat others with dignity, expect it in return)
- *Fidelidad* (loyalty)

Examples of traditional Latino/a gender roles

- **Machismo:** Actions or attitudes considered appropriate for males. Some behaviors include: Hard working, brave, tough, chivalrous (e.g., takes care of women/girls), good manners, and virile (strong and power-ful). In this role, the male must take care of his family and command the respect of others (Santiago-Rivera, Arredondo, & Gallardo-Cooper, 2002). The modern, exaggerated interpretation of machismo is often negative, including a man that drinks too much alcohol and who is sexist/chauvinistic.
  Machismo: Acciones o actitudes consideradas apropiadas para el género masculino. Algunos comportamientos incluyen: el trabajar duro, ser fuerte, ser valiente, ser caballeroso (p. ej. cuidar de las mujeres/las niñas), tener buenos modales y ser viril (fuerte y poderoso). En este papel, el hombre debe cuidar de su familia e imponer el respecto de otros. La interpretación moderna del machismo es muchas veces negativa, incluyendo a un hombre que toma mucho alcohol y que es un chovinista/sexista.

■ **Marianismo:** Tied to religion and the image of the Virgin Mary, who embodies a specific concept. A woman is expected to reflect traits of the Virgin Mary that include: pure, long-suffering, pious (good, moral, devout, dutiful), nurturing (takes care of others), self-sacrificing/other-centered. She also must be virtuous, humble, and spiritually strong.

Marianismo: Relacionado a la religión y a la imagen de la Virgen María, quien encarna un concepto específico. A una mujer se le espera reflejar estas características de la Virgen María que incluyen: la pureza, el sufrimiento, la piedad (la moralidad, la devoción, la diligencia), cuidar de otros, sacrificarse y preocuparse por otros. También debe ser virtuosa, humilde, y tener una firmeza espiritual.

Example Scenarios

- **Scenario #1:** You are being pressured by a friend to go to a party where you know there will be drugs and perhaps fighting. You do not feel comfortable with this, but you also don't want to say no to your friend.

  Un amigo te presiona para que vayas a una fiesta donde tú sabes que habrán drogas y quizás hasta algunas peleas. Tú no te sientes bien con la idea, pero a la misma vez no quieres decirle que no a tu amigo.

- **Scenario #2:** When walking down the hall at school you hear some kids talking about going to college. You overhear one of them mention a friend of yours, saying, "José? Forget it, everyone knows Latino/as aren't interested in going to college."

  Mientras caminas en los pasillos de la escuela oyes algunos muchachos hablar sobre el tema de asistir a la Universidad. Escuchas a uno de ellos mencionar a uno de tus amigos diciendo, "¿José? Olvídate, todos saben que a los Latino/as no les interesa asistir a la universidad."

- **Scenario #3:** You notice that your school counselor ignores the wishes of many Latino/a group members to go on to college—she often recommends they do not go, if they ask about it. You suspect she believes Latino/a group members are not as capable or do not desire a college education. During your appointment with her, she recommends that you go to a local trade school to learn welding, saying that it's an easy job for people who do not know English well. You want to go to college, not weld! You suspect she has stereotyped Latino/as and their abilities.

  Notas que tu consejero escolar ignora los deseos de varios miembros Latino/as de asistir a la Universidad y si ellos se lo piden ella les recomienda que ellos no asistan. Tú sospechas que ella cree que los miembros Latino/as del grupo no son capaces o no desean obtener una educación universitaria. Durante tu cita, ella te recomienda que tú vayas a una escuela de comercio para aprender soldadura, diciéndote que es un trabajo fácil para las personas que no saben un buen inglés. Tú quieres asistir a la universidad, y no aprender a soldar. Tú sospechas que ella tiene un estereotipo en lo que refiere a las habilidades de los Latino/as.

- **Scenario #4:** You notice every time you go into one of your local stores, one of the White teenagers working there always talks very slowly, loudly, and in a negative tone of voice to customers who are Latino/as, as if she thinks they don't speak English (even though most of them do). She is not as kind to those customers, either.

Te das cuenta que cada vez que entras a una de tus tiendas locales, uno de los jóvenes 'blancos' que trabaja allí siempre habla muy despacio, en voz alta, y en un tono negativo a los clientes que son Latino/as, como si ella pensara que ellos no hablan inglés (aunque la mayoría de ellos sí lo hablan). Ella tampoco los trata con amabilidad.

CHAPTER 5

LATINO/A YOUTH AND GRIEF

Mary G. Mayorga, Katrina Cook,
Tamara Hinojosa, Suzanne Mudge,
and Elizabeth A. Wardle

SESSION 1: MY RIGHT TO GRIEVE

Session Goal: To learn about the many ways people mourn/grieve.

Time Needed: 30–45 minutes

Suggested Group Size: 2–15

Materials Needed:

- A handout of the Six Basic Principles of Grief (Appendix E)
- Create and hang up each one of the Bill of Rights for Grieving (Appendix F)
- Blank paper, hung on the walls

Session Directions:

- Explain that everyone grieves differently, but that sometimes, people feel pressure to feel or act in certain ways. Explore how this may have been true for members.
- Hand out, review, and discuss the Six Basic Principles of Grief (Appendix E).
- When done, ask members to walk around the room and read the posted statements, which you can explain is a Bill of Rights for Grieving, written by a group of teenagers.

■ Afterward, elicit questions about rights that are unclear to them—which ones are confusing, or are new concepts? Encourage the members to explain to one another, and add your own age and culture-appropriate examples to further clarify.

Process Questions:

1. How was it for you to read the statements on the wall?
   ¿Cómo te sentiste al leer las frases de la pared?

2. Which right, or rights, were most important to you, and how so?
   ¿Cuál(es) derecho(s) fueron los más importantes para ti, en qué sentido?

3. Were there any you disagreed with or didn't like?
   ¿Hubieron algunos con los que tú estuviste en desacuerdo o que no te gustaron?

4. There is no right or wrong way to grieve, but sometimes we get a lot of pressure to grieve in certain ways—have you experienced that?
   No hay una manera correcta de expresar tu dolor, pero a veces sentimos presión de otras personas de expresar nuestro dolor de cierta manera. ¿Has tenido esta experiencia?

5. Do you sometimes think your loved ones should be grieving a certain way, but they're not?
   ¿A veces piensas que tus seres queridos deberían de expresar su dolor de cierta manera, pero no lo hacen?

6. How have you used Latino/a values and beliefs to help you deal with your grief?
   ¿Cómo has usado tus valores y creencias Latinas para ayudarte a enfrentar tu dolor?

7. Support systems are important in Latino/a cultures. Describe how your cultural support system has been helpful to you during this time.
   Los sistemas de apoyo son importantes en la cultura Latina. Describe cómo tus sistemas de apoyo te han ayudado durante este tiempo.

8. These rights were a few ideas created by some teenagers, but we have some blank paper on the walls to fill in—so what rights would you add that they didn't name?
   Estos derechos fueron productos de unas ideas creadas por algunos adolescentes, pero tenemos papel blanco en la pared para escribir—¿Cuáles de los derechos no mencionados añadirías?

SESSION 2: SHARED GRIEF

Session Goal: To gain understanding of the shared and common experiences of loss.

Time Needed: 30–45 minutes

Suggested Group Size: 2–15

Materials Needed:

- A picture book about grief, such as Sandra Cisneros' book for young adults, *Have You Seen Marie?* (2012)
- Writing utensils
- Blank paper for optional group step of writing their own grief story

Session Directions:

- Read all, or selected parts, of the book *Have You Seen Marie?* out loud to the group members, stopping to show the pictures.
- Process with the below questions.
- If time, prompt members to write their own brief stories, or to express their grief in other creative ways (poems, songs, pictures, comic strips). Allow them to share and process what was meaningful.

Process Questions:

1. What stood out to you about the story?
   ¿Qué se destacó para ti en el cuento?

2. Why do you think Sandra chose to help Roz search for Marie?
   ¿Por qué crees que Sandra decidió ayudar a Roz a buscar a Marie?

3. How did helping Roz search for Marie remind Sandra of her mother's death?
   ¿En qué manera al ayudar a Roz, le recordó a Sandra sobre la muerte de su madre?

4. What do you think Sandra means when she says she felt alone "like a glove left at a bus station?" And are there times when you have felt alone like that?
   ¿Qué tú crees significan las palabras de Sandra cuando ella dice que se sintió sola "como un guante olvidado en una estación de autobús?"

5. As Sandra and Roz asked neighbors if they had seen Marie, they discovered that many of them also experienced loss. What kinds of loss did different neighbors experience? (Possible answers include: family, friends, pets, health, or home.)
    Cuando Sandra y Roz le preguntaron a los vecinos si ellos habían visto a Marie, ellas descubrieron que muchos de ellos también habían sufrido una pérdida. ¿Qué clase de pérdida habían sufrido los vecinos? (Posibles respuestas incluyen: familiares, amigos, mascotas, la salud, o el hogar.)

6. How is your own grieving similar to, or different from, what she wrote in the story?
    ¿En qué asemeja o es diferente la manera como muestras tu duelo a lo que ella escribió en el cuento?

7. If you wrote your own grieving story, what would it be like? (If time allows, have them actually share afterward with one peer or the group, if comfortable.)
    Si tú escribieras tu propio cuento de duelo, ¿cómo sería? (si hay tiempo, hagan que ellos compartan sus respuestas con un miembro del grupo o con todo el grupo si se sienten a gusto).

8. Share with the rest of the group the loss you are experiencing right now.
    Comparte con el resto del grupo la pérdida que estás sufriendo en este momento.

SESSION 3: ARTISTIC EXPRESSION OF MY GRIEF

Session Goal: To express feelings of grief through creating a mandala.

Time Needed: 30–45 minutes

Suggested Group Size: 2–15

Materials Needed:

- Green, red, blue, purple/violet, yellow, black, and white construction paper
- Green, red, blue, purple/violet, yellow, black, and white crayons or markers
- Several round paper plates, to be used as a template for creating a mandala (if time is limited, the facilitator can have copies of different types of mandalas that each member can choose to color)
- A completed mandala, to show to the group as an example

Session Directions:

- Describe what a mandala is (Appendix G) and instruct the group members on how to construct it.
- Give a brief explanation of the colors (Appendix H) available for coloring the mandala.
- Each group member should choose a piece of construction paper.
- Give them approximately 20 minutes to draw and color the mandala.
- Once completed, have them share their mandalas and process the experience.

Process Questions:

1. How was this activity for you?
   ¿Qué te pareció esta actividad?

2. Talk about the feelings that your mandala represents for you.
   Habla sobre los sentimientos que para ti representa la mandala.

3. Describe to the group how the color(s) that you have chosen for your mandala define your grief.
   Descríbele al grupo cómo el color o los colores que escogiste para hacer tu mandala define(n) tu pena.

4. Describe to the group your reasons for choosing the color(s) for making your mandala.
   Descríbele al grupo las razones por las cuales escogiste el color o los colores para hacer tu mandala.

5. In what ways does your culture encourage you to wear certain colors when you are grieving?

   ¿En qué manera tu cultura te impulsa a usar ciertos colores cuando estás de duelo?

6. Are there any other colors you might use that haven't been mentioned, and what might they mean?

   ¿Existen otros colores que usarías que no se han mencionado, que significarían ellos?

7. What is most important from today that you will remember or use?

   ¿Qué sería lo más importante del día de hoy que recordarás o utilizarás?

SESSION 4: BOLSILLO DE UN REQUERDO

Session Goal: Creating a 'memory' pocket representative of the deceased love one.

Time Needed: 30–45 minutes

Suggested Group Size: 2–15

Materials Needed:

- Various colors of construction paper
- Tape/glue
- Stapler
- Markers/colored pencils/crayons
- Writing utensils

Session Directions:

- Note that, in the Latino/a culture, having a place to honor the deceased is very important. Explain that you will each create a *bolsillo* or small bag that can hold a small picture or memento of their loved one.
- Give a brief description of how to make a *bolsillo* using construction paper (Appendix I).
- Allow approximately 20 minutes to make their creations.
- Afterwards, process the activity.

Process Questions:

1. What item will you choose to go into your *bolsillo*?
   ¿Qué artículo pondrías en tu bolsillo?

2. What are your reasons for choosing this item to place into your *bolsillo*?
   ¿Cuáles son tus razones por escoger este artículo para poner en tu bolsillo?

3. How does this item honor and show respect for your loved one?
   ¿Cómo muestra este artículo honor y respeto hacía tu ser querido?

4. As noted earlier, in the Latino/a culture, having a place of honor for the deceased is very important. Is this true for your family, and how so?
   ¿Cómo se notó anteriormente, en la cultura Latina, tener un lugar para dar honor al difunto es muy importante? ¿Es esto cierto en tu familia, cómo lo es?

5. Where will you keep your *bolsillo*?
   ¿Dónde vas a guardar tu bolsillo?

6. Will you share it with anyone?

   ¿Lo vas a compartir con alguien?

7. How did this activity help you remember and honor your loved one?

   ¿Cómo te ayudó esta actividad a recordar y a honrar a tu ser querido?

SESSION 5: OJO DE DIOS (GOD'S EYE)

Session Goal: Creating an Ojo de Dios as a tangible symbol of their love for a lost one.

Time Needed: 30–45 minutes

Suggested Group Size: 2–15

Materials Needed:

- Handout, one for each student, with the instructions on how to make an Ojo de Dios (Appendix J)
- Two popsicle sticks for each participant
- Several rolls of yarn (various colors)
- Tape/glue
- Poster board/foam board

Session Directions:

- Introduce the concept of the Ojo de Dios by saying the following:
- "The Ojo de Dios is a simple weaving made across two or more sticks. The origin is credited to the Huichol Indians of Jalisco, Mexico and they symbolized the ability to see and understand things that are unknown and the unknowable. Over time, many people came to think of the Ojo de Dios symbol as representing God looking down on them with love. For today's activity, the symbol of Ojo de Dios will represent how each of you looks with love on the person you lost."
- Demonstrate to members how to make an Ojo de Dios (Appendix J).
- Ask members to create their own unique Ojo de Dios in honor of the person they are grieving.
- Ask members to share their project with one another or with the entire group (depending on comfort level), using process questions below.
- With their permission, place completed projects together on a large poster board, which the facilitator can then bring to future sessions as a reminder of their loved ones.

Process Questions:

1. Tell me, what was it like for you to create your Ojo de Dios?
   ¿Dime cómo te sentiste al crear tu Ojo de Dios?
2. What is the significance of the colors of yarn you chose?
   ¿Cuál es el significado de los colores del hilo que escogiste?

3. How does this Ojo de Dios represent the person you loved who has died?
   ¿Cómo representa este Ojo de Dios a tu ser querido que ha fallecido?

4. What is your reaction to other group members as they talked about their Ojo de Dios and the person they loved who has died?
   ¿Cuál es tu reacción hacia los otros miembros del grupo cuando ellos hablaron sobre su Ojo de Dios y del ser querido que había muerto?

5. What do you think about when you look at your Ojo de Dios?
   ¿En qué piensas cuando miras a tu Ojo de Dios?

6. What is most important to you about today's session?
   ¿Qué fue lo más importante sobre la sesión de hoy?

Facilitator Notes: You could also allow group members to take their craft home and encourage them to hang them in a meaningful location.

SESSION 6: *CONSEJOS*

Session Goal: Reflection about *consejos*, or words of wisdom, that their deceased loved one may have wanted to tell them, but did not get a chance to.

Time Needed: 30–45 minutes

Suggested Group Size: 2–15

Materials Needed:

- Blank paper
- Markers/colored pencils/crayons
- Writing utensils
- Glue
- Ribbon
- Craft materials, as desired (glitter, feathers, macaroni, pipe cleaners, etc.)

Session Directions:

- Ask group members to reflect on how their loved one who has died influenced their lives, as well as how they may have influenced their loved one. Encourage members to describe important and inspiring moments that they shared with their loved one.
- Next, explain that *consejos* are like words of wisdom or pieces of advice that are encouraging and supportive. Ask group members to imagine the *consejos* their loved one may have wanted to give them, but did not get a chance to. These *consejos* may be things their loved one had already said or may not have found the opportunity to express. They may include advice, gratitude, and words of support.
- Provide a sheet of paper to each group member and ask them to express these *consejos* in writing or illustration using the materials provided. Group members are encouraged to write in whichever language they feel most comfortable.
- After group members have finished creating their *consejos*, invite them to read them to the group (if comfortable) or to show and describe their illustrations.
- Process the experience with the below questions.
- After all members have shared, provide each with a ribbon so that they can roll their paper into a scroll. This represents a symbolic sense of closure.

Process Questions:

1. What emotions came up for you while creating or sharing your *consejos*?
   ¿Cuáles emociones sentiste mientras creabas o compartías tus consejos?

2. What reactions do you have to the *consejos* that were just shared?
   ¿Cuáles son tus reacciones a los consejos que se acaban de compartir?

3. What words and illustrations stood out to you the most?
   ¿Para ti, cuáles palabras e ilustraciones se destacaron más?

4. Were there any comments that stood out to you?
   ¿Para ti, hubieron algunos comentarios que se destacaron?

5. What will you do with your *consejos* after today?
   ¿Qué harás con tus consejos después del día de hoy?

6. How will your *consejos* influence you as you move forward in life?
   ¿Cómo te van a influir tus consejos al seguir adelante en la vida?

7. How does hearing these *consejos* make you feel closer as a group?
   ¿En que forma escuchando estos consejos te hace sentir más conectado al grupo?

REFERENCES

Cisneros, S. (2012). *Have you seen Marie?* New York, NY: Knopf Doubleday Publishing Group.

The Dougy Center Teens (n.d.). *The bill of rights of grieving teens.* Retrieved from http://www.dougy.org/grief-resources/bill-of-rights/

The Dougy Center (n.d.). *Six basic principles of teen grief.* Retrieved from http://www.dougy.org/grief-resources/how-to-help-a-grieving-teen/

McArdle, T. (n.d.). *How to draw a mandala.* Retrieved from http://www.art-is-fun.com/how-to-draw-a-mandala.html

Six Basic Principles of Teen Grief

*Adapted from Helping Teens Cope with Death, The Dougy Center

Principle #1: Sometimes, when we have lost a loved one, we have a hard time with our emotions. We may feel sad, frightened, or angry. We may not know how to let others know what we are feeling. Sometimes, we are told not to feel the things we are feeling.

Principio #1: A veces, cuando hemos perdido a un ser querido, tenemos dificultad de expresar nuestras emociones. Nos podemos sentir tristes, con miedo, o enojados. Quizás no sabemos expresarle a otros nuestros sentimientos. A veces, nos dicen que no debemos sentir lo que estamos sintiendo.

Principle #2: Everyone expresses their feelings differently when grieving and there is no right or wrong way to do this.

Principio #2: Todos expresan sus emociones de una manera diferente cuando están en duelo y no hay una manera correcta o incorrecta de hacerlo.

Principle #3: We can decide how to best express our feelings, such as talking with someone, writing in a journal, or drawing a picture that shows how we feel.

Principio #3: Podemos decidir cuál es la mejor manera de expresar nuestros sentimientos, como hablar con alguien, escribir en un cuaderno, o dibujar una imagen que muestre la manera que nos sentimos.

Principle #4: My feelings about the loss of my loved one will be different from other people's feelings.

Principio #4: Mis sentimientos sobre la pérdida de mi ser querido serán diferente a los sentimientos de otras personas.

Principle #5: It is important to have someone to talk to when you have lost a loved one (a friend, family member, teacher, or school counselor).

Principio #5: Es importante tener a alguien con quién hablar cuando has perdido a un ser querido (un amigo, un familiar, un maestro o un consejero de la escuela).

Principle #6: Remember that you will always miss your loved one, but over time, the loss will feel less painful, and you will learn how to get through that loss.

Principio #6: Recuerda que siempre extrañarás a tu ser querido, pero con el tiempo, la pérdida será menos dolorosa, y tú aprenderás a superar esa pérdida.

The Bill of Rights for Grieving

*Adapted from Teens at the Dougy Center

You have the right:	***Tú tienes el derecho:***
. . . to have your questions answered honestly	*. . . de tener respuestas honestas a tus preguntas*
. . . to have someone listen to you and how you feel	*. . . de tener a alguien que te escuche y comprenda como te sientes*
. . . to not talk about the loss until you are ready	*. . . de no hablar de la pérdida hasta que estés listo*
. . . to visit the place where the person died	*. . . de visitar el lugar dónde la persona murió*
. . . to express how you are feeling as long as it does not hurt you physically	*. . . de expresar tus sentimientos siempre que no te haga daño fisicamente*
. . . to have the feelings you are having	*. . . de sentirte como te sientes*
. . . to be angry about the loss	*. . . de sentir ira sobre tu pérdida*
. . . to ask your family about the funeral	*. . . de preguntarle a tu familia sobre el entierro*
. . . to find ways to grieve that help you	*. . . de encontrar maneras de expresar tu pena que te ayuden*

What is a Mandala?

A mandala is an abstract design that is usually circular in form and can be either a complex or simple design. The word mandala is a 'Sanskrit' word that means 'circle.' Mandalas represent the connection between our inner worlds and outer realities. They can contain geometric forms and images that carry meaning for the person who is creating the mandala. Designing your own mandala can be both inspirational and therapeutic. When you design a mandala you have the freedom to use your creativity to create a mandala drawing that is uniquely yours (McArdle, n.d.).

INSTRUCTIONS FOR DRAWING A MANDALA:

1. Use a circle template (a paper dinner plate works well) and a large piece of blank paper (construction paper or a white sheet of paper). A mandala can be 8" to 10" in diameter.
2. Make a light pencil outline of the circle template on the paper.
3. Use markers or color pencils to make your mandala. Pick a color that you are drawn to and begin to make marks on the paper.
4. Take a deep breath, relax, and clear your mind of any concerns. Create your mandala by filling the circle with lines, shapes, and colors. It is not necessary to stay or even begin the drawing within the lines of the circle.
5. When you have completed the drawing, you may want to give it a title. You may want to date the mandala drawing.

APPENDIX H: SESSION 3: ARTISTIC EXPRESSION OF MY GRIEF

Colors in Latino/a Culture

Green is representative of death
Red is representative of danger or success
Blue is representative of trouble
Purple/violet or yellow is representative of mourning
Black is representative of mourning
White is representative of religion

Verde representa la muerte
Rojo representa el peligro o el éxito
Azul representa los problemas
Morado/violeta o el amarillo representa el duelo
Negro representa el duelo
Blanco representa la religión

Instructions for Making a Bolsillo

1. Start with a sheet of construction paper.
2. Fold the construction paper in half (length-wise first).
3. Fold the length-wise construction paper in half.
4. This will create a square pocket.
5. Create a small 'lip' on each open-ended section of the pocket to give it a finished look.
6. You are now ready to either glue or staple the ends together to give you a *bolsillo* in which you can put your memento.
7. Once you have glued or stapled your *bolsillo* together, you are ready to decorate it.

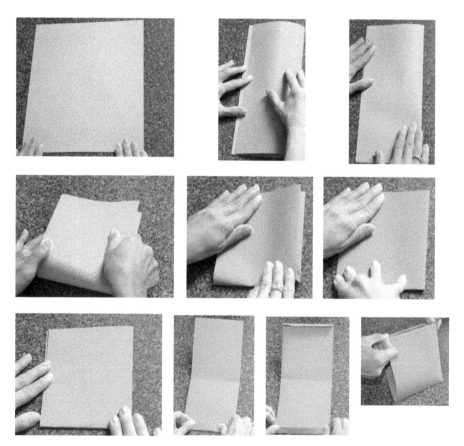

Figures 5.1–5.10 Making a Bolsillo

How to Make an Ojo de Dios

1. Glue two sticks together in the shape of a cross. The points of the cross are numbered for reference in the directions. You will not be numbering your sticks.
2. Take the end of the yarn and lay it across the center of the cross, leaving a tail of about 2"–3". As you wrap the yarn, the tail will be wrapped with the stick so that it will not be observable. Pull the yarn behind stick number 1 as close to the center as possible.
3. From the back, wrap the yarn completely around stick 1 as close to the center as possible. Then, wrap it underneath stick 2.
4. Wrap it completely around stick 2.
5. Repeat wrapping around the sticks for sticks 3 and 4. Then, go to stick 1 again and continue wrapping around each stick until the Ojo de Dios is the size you want. Cut the yarn about 3" away from the Ojo de Dios and wrap the remaining loose yarn underneath the yarn of your Ojo de Dios so it isn't seen.
6. The completed Ojo de Dios will look like this.

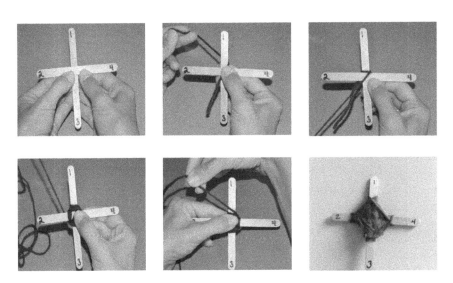

Figures 5.11–5.16 Making an Ojo de Dois

CHAPTER
6

UNDERSTANDING LGBTQIA LATINO/A YOUTH

Kara Ieva and Kristina Weiss

SESSION 1: CONSTELLATION OF STARS

Session Goal: Identify where group members are in their coming out and identity process.

Time Needed: 30–45 minutes

Suggested Group Size: 2–15

Materials Needed:

- One large, pre-cut star for each group member
- Markers/colored pencils/crayons
- Writing utensils

Session Directions:

- Identify group purpose and allow members to choose several rules for the group.
- Give each member a pre-cut star.
- Instruct members to write the following on different points of their star (they may need two per point): name; various social and gender identities (e.g., race, ethnicity, religion, gender, sexual orientation); interests; important family members; role models.

- Once stars are completed, have them share and explain to the entire group.
- Process the meaning of the activity with the below questions.
- Before closing, explain that when all stars are put together, they create a constellation. Each is bright and unique on its own, yet together they create a strong unity in the sky, just as the group itself creates a wholeness and a particular beauty together.

Process Questions:

1. Which star point is the most meaningful to you?
   De los puntos que escribiste en la estrella, ¿Cuál tiene más significado para ti?

2. When listing your family members, how did you decide who to list?
   ¿Cómo decidiste a quién de los miembros de tu familia incluir en la lista?

3. Why did you choose your role model? Is your role model of the same ethnicity as you?
   ¿Por qué escogiste tu modelo a seguir? ¿Es tú modelo a seguir de tu misma raza étnica?

4. What values does this role model possess?
   ¿Cuáles valores posee tu modelo a seguir?

5. What message do they send about being female or male?
   ¿Qué mensaje envían sobre ser masculino o femenino?

6. Are the messages sent by your role model consistent with Latino/a cultural beliefs?
   ¿Los mensajes que muestran tus modelos a seguir son uniformes con las creencias de la cultura Latina?

7. How do some points on your star influence or interact with others (such as how does your race or ethnicity influence or interact with your sexual orientation)?
   ¿Cómo los puntos de tu estrella interactúan el uno al otro (por ejemplo, cómo tu raza o etnicidad influye tu orientación sexual)?

8. How do all the points of your star reflect aspects of your Latino/a culture?
   ¿Cómo reflejan los puntos de tu estrella los aspectos de tu cultura Latina?

SESSION 2: NAVIGATING THE STARS

Session Goal: To learn common vocabulary and labels used within the LGBTQIA community.

Time Needed: 30–45 minutes

Suggested Group Size: 2–15

Materials Needed:

- Whiteboard or large writing paper
- Markers/colored pencils/crayons
- Writing utensils
- Tape/glue
- Common Vocabulary Handout (Appendix K)

Session Directions:

- Before group begins:

  - Write vocabulary terms (Appendix K) on separate pieces of paper and tape each piece of paper onto the walls, spaced around the room.
  - Create a page of definitions of terms, pre-cut (each definition separate from the other). One set for each group member.

- Introduce the group topic, and hand out the pre-cut definitions to each group member. Instruct members to walk around the room and tape definitions they were provided to what they believe is the appropriate vocabulary word.
- Once completed, review and discuss, using the below process questions.

Process Questions:

1. Do you agree or disagree with certain vocabulary words and definitions?
   ¿Estás de acuerdo o en desacuerto con ciertas palabras de vocabulario y definiciones?

2. What most stood out to you? Which one(s) do you have questions about?
   ¿Qué se destacó más para ti? ¿Tienes alguna pregunta sobre alguna de ellas?

3. Which words do you feel most connected to?
   ¿Con cuáles palabras te sientes más conectado/a?

4. Were there terminologies that surprised you?
   ¿Cuáles palabras te sorprendieron?

5. Within the Latino/a community, are there particular terms or slang used when referring to people in the **LGBTQA** community? Which of these terms or slang are positive, negative?

   ¿Dentro de la comunidad Latina, existen algunas palabras en particular que se refieren a personas de la comunidad LGBTQA? ¿Cuáles de estas palabras son positivas? ¿Cuáles son negativas?

6. Do the terms or slang used within the Latino/a culture match or differ from the vocabulary list when identifying the **LGBTQA** community?

   ¿Son iguales o diferentes las palabras usadas en la cultura Latina a la lista de palabras que identifican a la comunidad LGBTQA?

7. Of all the terms discussed, what three stand out as your own identification within the **LGBTQA** and Latino/a community?

   De los términos discutidos, nombra tres que se destacan en tu propia identificación con la comunidad LGBTQA y Latina.

8. Are these identifications you feel comfortable sharing with others?

   ¿Te sientes a gusto compartiendo estas identificaciones con otras personas?

SESSION 3: GRAVITATIONAL PULL: WHAT INFLUENCES US

Session Goal: Identify who has influenced members' gender identities and sexual orientation.

Time Needed: 30–45 minutes

Suggested Group Size: 2–15

Materials Needed:

- Construction paper
- Markers/colored pencils/crayons
- Writing utensils
- Tape/glue
- 10–15 magazines (current, pop culture, age appropriate, Latino/a influenced)

Session Directions:

- Begin by asking members to identify and explain certain identities that are most important to them, offering examples (e.g., gender, sexual orientation, and ethnicity).
- Ask them to identify persons from the media and pop culture who have most influenced those identities, both positively and negatively.
- Instruct members to use the magazines and creativity with drawings, symbols, etc., to create a collage of how different influences (e.g., media, Latino/a culture, family, religion, etc.) have impacted their gender identity and sexual orientation.
- Once members have completed their collages, reconvene and share with one another.

Process Questions:

1. Are there any influences that overlap in areas of group members' lives?
   ¿Hay algunas influencias que coinciden en parte en las vidas de los miembros del grupo?

2. Which influences have assisted in their gender or sexual identity?
   ¿Cuáles influencias han ayudado a su identidad sexual o de género?

3. Are there influences that have negatively impacted their view of their own sexual or gender identity?
   ¿Hay influencias que han impactado negativamente el punto de vista sobre su propia identidad sexual o de género?

4. Who or what is a large influence in your life?
   ¿Quién o qué es la influencia más importante en tu vida?

5. How do certain influences impact more in one area in your life than in another?
   ¿Cómo ciertas influencias impactan más en un área de tu vida que en otra?

6. What are the main themes within each group member's collage?
   ¿Cuáles son los temas más importantes en el collage de cada miembro?

7. How do any of these influences impact how you display your sexual orientation or gender identity?
   ¿Cómo estas influencias impactan la manera como tú muestras tu sexualidad o tu identidad de género?

8. What areas do you feel are more influenced than others?
   ¿Cuáles áreas sientes tú influyen más que otras?

SESSION 4: MAGNITUDE OF THE STARS: INTERSECTION OF SEXUALITY AND ETHNICITY

Session Goal: Critically explore the intersection of sexuality and ethnicity.

Time Needed: 30–45 minutes

Suggested Group Size: 2–15

Materials Needed:

- Blank paper, two pieces per group member
- Markers/colored pencils/crayons
- Writing utensils
- Tape/glue

Session Directions:

- Ask members if they know the definition of ethnicity (if not, provide one, such as "one's culture, the language you speak, your food, values, traditions").
- Explore members' sense of ethnicity—how it developed, how strong it is, how it may influence their lifestyle and decisions.
- Give group members two pieces of paper, and explain that society and our communities create labels that stigmatize particular groups of people. Ask group members to think of a label that their ethnicity has created for those within the LGBTQIA community or that they are currently faced with due to their ethnicity and sexuality. If group members have trouble thinking of labels, brainstorm as a group labels they may have heard.
- Instruct group members to write a label on one of the pieces of paper. They will then tape the paper to themselves, allowing their peers to see the label.
- Group facilitators should discuss labels and their meanings with group members.
- Suggest that labels are only as impactful as we allow them to be. Emphasize that individuals have a choice to define themselves.
- Ask members to remove their labels and invite them to destroy them by ripping them up, if they find their label hurtful/harmful.
- Instruct group members to use a second piece of paper to create a new label, with a definition, that truly describes who they are. Have them tape the label to themselves.

Process Questions:

1. How did it feel to destroy the negative label?
    ¿Cómo te sentiste al destruír la etiqueta negativa?

2. Did any members visualize or say anything in their head while destroying the label?
    ¿Algunos de los miembros del grupo pensó en alguna cosa mientras destruían la etiqueta?

3. How can group members destroy hurtful labels in their lives?
    ¿Cómo pueden los miembros del grupo destruir las etiquetas ofensivas en sus vidas?

4. Are there labels about LGBTQIA within the Latino/a community you would like to destroy?
    ¿Existen etiquetas sobre LGBTQIA dentro de la comunidad Latina que quisieran destruir?

5. How does your new label identify you?
    ¿Cómo te identifica la nueva etiqueta?

6. How can you begin to live with the new label?
    ¿Cómo podrías empezar a vivir con la nueva etiqueta?

7. What is most important about today that you will take with you?
    ¿Qué es lo más importante sobre el día de hoy que llevarás contigo?

SESSION 5: SHINING THE LIGHT WITHIN

Session Goal: Discuss the coming-out process.

Time Needed: 30–45 minutes

Suggested Group Size: 2–15

Materials Needed:

- Poem, *Colors* by Pwnorton (Appendix L), one copy for each member
- Blank paper
- Markers/colored pencils/crayons
- Writing utensils

Session Directions:

- Explain the purpose of that day's session, and hand out copies of the poem, *Colors* (Appendix L), to each group member.
- Ask one member to read the poem in English, and another in Spanish.
- Explore reactions to the poems, in relation to 'coming out' and the different colors.
- Ask members to discuss their current process of disclosing their sexual orientation or gender identity to others. Have members who are comfortable share their experiences.
- Give a piece of paper to each group member and ask them to write their own coming-out story (if they do not have one, they can imagine what it might be). Stress this can be a story or creative poems, a rap song, or can include pictures. See facilitator notes on this.
- Once completed, ask those who are comfortable to briefly share (or use dyads).

Process Questions:

1. How did it feel to write your stories?
   ¿Qué se sintieron al escribir sus historias?

2. How did it feel to tell your story to someone else?
   ¿Cómo te sentiste al compartir tu historia con otra persona?

3. Was your story true or what you are hoping will happen?
   ¿Fue verdadera tu historia o fue un producto de lo que tú esperabas que ocurriera?

4. What parts of your story do you think will happen?
   ¿Cuáles partes de tu historia crees tú van a ocurrir?

5. Why did you choose particular individuals to be in your story?
   ¿Por qué escogiste a ciertas personas para que tomaran parte en tu historia?

6. Why did you choose that particular way to come out, in your story?
   En tu historia, ¿Por qué escogiste esa manera particular de revelarte/descubrirte?

7. What is the most important thing you will take away with you from today's session on 'coming out'?
   ¿Qué es lo más importante que llevarás contigo de la sesión de hoy sobre el proceso de 'revelación y descubrimiento'?

Facilitator Notes: For safety and confidentiality reasons, facilitators may want to have members share their stories verbally. If members do write their stories, consider asking members to destroy them afterward.

SESSION 6: SUPPORT IN THE STARS

Session Goal: Identify strategies for coping with societal bias toward LGBTQIA members.

Time Needed: 30–45 minutes

Suggested Group Size: 2–15

Materials Needed:

- Handout with national LGBTQIA support groups (Appendix M) (possibly add your own local support groups to this)
- Four index cards per group member
- Markers/colored pencils/crayons
- Writing utensils
- Two bags, large enough for index cards, one labeled 'on my own' and the other, 'together'
- Small pebbles or marbles (four per group member)

Session Directions:

- Give each group member four index cards.
- Instruct members to anonymously identify and list their main concerns, one per index card, for coming out and openly living as a Latino/a LGBTQIA member.
- Ask members to place the cards into the bag labeled 'on my own.' Note that they will review them later.
- Point to the bag labeled 'on my own' and explain that, when individuals have problems, they may choose (or be forced) to face their problems alone.
- Ask members to identify how they have dealt with various types of stressors in their lives (i.e., school, work, family issues, friendships, relationships, peer pressure), ultimately relating this to ways they can deal with LGBTQIA-related stressors.
- Discuss and address the common issues and concerns of LGBTQIA bullying and discrimination, along with addressing their rights. Remind them that if they reach out for help, others can help them resolve or cope with a problem.
- Take turns having members pull an index card from the bag and read the card out loud. Then, as a group, brainstorm various coping skills and supports that can be used for that issue.

- After each card is discussed, the group member who read the index card will place the card into the bag marked 'together.'
- Once completed with all the cards, state that the 'together' bag is now full and stress that they are all in this together. When individuals reach out and ask for help, they can all support one another and face challenges together.

Process Questions:

1. Of the concerns discussed today about the coming-out process, which do you share with others?
   De los asuntos discutidos hoy sobre el proceso de 'revelación,' ¿Qué inquietudes compartes con otros?

2. In what areas of your life do you feel you can best use these coping skills?
   ¿En cuáles áreas de tu vida sientes que puedes emplear estas estrategias?

3. Which coping skill do you feel may be most useful to you?
   ¿Cuál estrategia de superación tú sientes puede ser la más útil para ti?

4. How can we support each other when we are going through the coming-out process?
   ¿Cómo nos podemos apoyar el uno al otro cuando estamos pasando por el proceso de 'revelación'?

5. Who are individuals in your life that you can go to when going through a difficult situation?
   ¿Con quién/es puedes contar cuando estás pasando por una situación difícil?

6. What about being Latino/a gives you strength and most helps you cope in relation to this topic?
   Sobre ser Latino, ¿Qué es lo que te da fuerza y más te ayuda en relación a este tema?

7. What do you want to take from today's session that is most meaningful to you?
   ¿Qué es lo más importante de la sesión de hoy que quieres llevar contigo?

Facilitator Notes: It is important to pay attention to any signs of member self-harm or suicidality, in relation to painful topics such as bullying. It is crucial that group facilitators address any emotions that may arise during this conversation and only return to the topic if all members are emotionally and psychologically able to continue. Facilitators should also be ready with resources related to referring youth in support for sexual harassment, bullying, self-harm/suicide, etc.

REFERENCES

Pwnorton (2008). *Coming out poem* [Web log message]. Retrieved from http://emptyclosets.com/forum/chit-chat/8376-coming-out-poem.html

Common Vocabulary Worksheet

Adapted from the Carleton College Gender and Sexuality Center LGBT Vocabulary 101 handout and the Ohio University Lesbian, Gay, Bisexual, Transgender Center, A Common Vocabulary pamphlet

Ally: A heterosexual or LGBTQIA person who supports LGBTQIA persons.
Aliado: Una persona heterosexual o LGBTQIA que apoya a la gente LGBTQIA.

Asexual: When a persons does not desire sexual intimacy with others.
Asexual: Cuando una persona no desea tener intimidad sexual con otros.

Bisexual: A person who is emotionally, physically, spiritually, and sexually attracted to members of more than one gender.
Bisexual: Una persona que esta emocional, física, espiritual, y sexualmente atraída a miembros de más de un género.

Coming Out: The life-long process of discovering, defining, and proclaiming one's own sexuality and gender identity to oneself, family, friends, and others.
Descubrirse/Revelarse: El proceso perpetuo de descubrimiento, definición y proclamación de identidad sexual propia y género de identidad a uno mismo, a la familia, a los amigos y a los demás.

Gay: A man whose primary romantic, emotional, physical, and sexual attractions are to other men. This term can also be used to apply to lesbians, bisexuals, and on some occasions, as an umbrella term for all LGBTQIA people.
Gay: Un hombre cuya atracción romántica, emocional, física y sexual primaria son hacia otro hombre. Esta palabra también puede aplicar a las lesbianas, a los bisexuales, y en algunas ocasiones, puede ser un término general para toda la población LGBTQIA.

Gender Identity/Expression: A person's sense of being masculine, feminine, or other gendered. This may or may not agree with the traditional societal gender roles outlined for their sex.
Género e Identidad de Expresión: El sentido de una persona de ser masculina, femenina, o de otro género. Esto puede o no puede estar de acuerdo con los roles de género tradicionales atribuidos a su sexo.

Genderfluid: A form of gender identity (what gender you feel like) that flows or mixes between boy and girl. Some days the person feels more like a boy, other days, a girl.

Fluidez de Género: Una forma de identificación de género que se mezcla entre hombre y mujer. Algunas veces, la persona se siente como un hombre y otras veces como una mujer.

Gender Role: The societal and cultural expectations of people based upon their biological sex.

Papel de Género: Las expectativas culturales y sociales de las personas basadas en su sexo biológico.

Heterosexual: A person who has emotional, physical, spiritual, and/or sexual attractions to persons of the opposite sex.

Heterosexual: Una persona que se siente atraída emocional, física, espiritual, y/o sexualmente a personas del sexo opuesto.

Homosexual: Attraction to persons of the same sex. Many prefer the terms 'gay' or 'lesbian' to describe their identities.

Homosexual: Atracción al mismo sexo. Muchos prefieren el término 'gay' o 'lesbiana' para describir su identidad.

Intersexual: A variety of physical conditions whereby a person has sexual or reproductive anatomy that is neither female or male.

Intersexual: Una variedad de condiciones físicas donde una persona tiene una anatomía reproductiva que no es ni femenina ni masculina.

Lesbian: A woman whose emotional, physical, and sexual attractions are to other women.

Lesbiana: Una mujer cuya atracción emocional, física y sexual es hacia otra mujer.

LGBTQIA: Lesbian, Gay, Bisexual, Transgender, Queer, Intersex, and Asexual.

LGBTQIA: Lesbiana, gay, bisexual, transgénero, queer, intersexual, y asexual.

Pride: Not being ashamed of oneself and/or showing one's pride to others by coming out, speaking out, marching, etc. Being open, honest, and comfortable.

Orgullo: No estar avergonzado de si mismo y mostrar nuestro orgullo a otras personas al revelarnos. Ser honesto y abierto.

Queer: Umbrella term, could mean anyone who identifies as LGBTQIA, or anyone who feels outside the norm related to gender expectations or roles.

Queer: Término general que puede referirse a cualquier persona que se identifica como LGBTQIA, o puede referirse a cualquiera que se siente fuera de la norma en cuanto a las expectativas de género.

Sex: Sex refers to one's physical state—e.g., gonads, hormones, internal reproductive organs. This does not indicate sexual orientation (e.g., who one is attracted to) or one's gender identity (e.g., internal sense of one's maleness, femaleness, or other) or gender expression (e.g., the way you behave/express yourself related to gender expectations).

Sexo: Refiriéndose al estado propio físico—p. ej. gónadas, hormonas, órganos de reproducción. Esto no indica la orientación sexual (p. ej. a quién uno se siente atraído, o la identidad de género (p. ej. El sentido interno de la masculinidad o feminidad u otro) o la expresión de género (p. ej. La manera en la cuál uno se comporta o se expresa en relación a las expectativas para cada género).

Sexual Orientation: How one thinks of oneself in terms of to whom one is sexually or romantically attracted. Orientation is not dependent on physical experience, but rather on a person's feelings and attractions.

Orientación sexual: Como uno piensa de si mismo en términos de a quién uno se siente atraído sexual y románticamente. La orientación no depende de la experiencia física sino en los sentimientos y atracciones de la persona.

Transgender: Used both as an umbrella term and as an identity. Broadly, it refers to those who do not identify or are uncomfortable with their assigned gender and gender roles. As an identity the term refers to anyone who transgresses traditional sex and gender categories.

Transgénero: Usado como ambos un término general y como identidad. Ampliamente, se refiere a esos quiénes no se identifican o se sienten incómodos con el género y roles de género asignado a ellos. Como identidad se refiere a cualquiera que sobrepasa las categorías tradicionales de sexo y género.

Transsexual: A person whose core gender identity is 'opposite' their assigned sex. Transsexuals may live as the opposite sex, undergo hormone therapy, and/or have sex reassignment surgery to 'match' their bodies with their gender identity.

Transexual: Una persona cuyo género de identidad principal es 'opuesto' a su asignado género. Los transexuales pueden vivir como el sexo opuesto, tomar hormonas de terapia, y/o tener una operación de reasignación de sexo para igualar a sus cuerpos con su identidad de género.

By Pwnorton

Reprinted with permission of http://emptyclosets.com/forum/chit-chat/8376-coming-out-poem.html administrators

Colors	*Colores*
I walk along this path	*Yo camino en este sendero*
Unknown to others,	*No conocido a otros,*
Newly discovered by me.	*Apenas descubierto por mi.*
And see the colors.	*Y veo los colores.*
They mingle with each other,	*Se mezclan el uno al otro,*
But not with those unlike them.	*Pero no con esos que no se asemejan a ellos.*
Blue with blue,	*El azul con el azul,*
Red with red,	*El rojo con el rojo,*
Green with green,	*El verde con el verde,*
Pink	*Rosado*
With pink.	*Con rosado.*
They are happy this way,	*Así son felices,*
Undisturbed	*Sin ser molestados*
By the constant bickering	*Por las constantes riñas*
Of the others who look in their direction,	*De otros que miran en su dirección,*
Pointing, laughing, making jokes.	*Señalando, riéndose, y burlándose.*
Blue is happy with blue.	*El azul es feliz con el azul.*
Red is happy with red.	*El rojo es feliz con el rojo.*
Green is happy with green.	*El verde es feliz con el verde.*
Pink	*Rosado*
Is happy with pink.	*Es feliz con el rosado.*
If this path were to be found,	*Si se encuentra este sendero,*
The colors would fade,	*Los colores perderían su intensidad,*
Not showing their true selves,	*No mostrarían quiénes son,*
For fear of being ridiculed,	*Por miedo a que se burlen de ellos,*
For fear of being laughed at.	*Por miedo a que se rían de ellos.*
So blue joins pink,	*Entonces el azul se une al rosado,*
Green with red.	*El verde al rojo.*
Constant pain of this mask,	*Un dolor constante de esta máscara*

Trying to please all,	*Tratando de complacer a todos,*
Not being what they were meant to be.	*Sin ser lo que debieron ser.*
But slowly, the colors separate.	*Pero lentamente los colores se separan.*
Blue joins blue,	*El azul se une al azul,*
Red joins red,	*El rojo se une al rojo,*
Green joins green,	*El verde se une al verde,*
Pink	*Rosado*
Joins pink.	*Se une al Rosado.*
The others point, laugh,	*Los otros señalan, se ríen,*
But the colors don't mind.	*Pero a los colores no les importa.*
They never apologize	*Ellos nunca piden disculpas*
For who they are.	*Por quiénes son.*
They never apologize	*Ellos nunca piden disculpas*
For being what the others hate,	*De ser lo que otros odian,*
For what makes themselves happy.	*Por lo que a ellos los hace ser feliz.*

List of National LGBTQ Organizations

PFLAG
PFLAG National Office
(202) 467-8180
http://community.pflag.org

Gay Alliance
(585) 244-8640
http://www.gayalliance.org

SGA
(415) 552-4229
http://www.gsanetwork.org

The Trevor Project
1-866-488-7386
http://www.thetrevorproject.org

Human Rights Campaign
(800) 777-4723
http://www.hrc.org

Center Link
(954) 765-6024
http://www.lgbtcenters.org

Stopbullying.gov
http://www.stopbullying.gov/index.html

CREANDO ESPERANZA: HOPE GROUPS

Lisa M. Edwards and Jessica B. McClintock

SESSION 1: INTRODUCTION TO HOPE MODEL

Session Goal: To learn the Hope Model and help members develop a personal goal for group.

Time Needed: 35–40 minutes

Suggested Group Size: 2–15

Materials Needed:

- Prior to the session, prepare a set of cutouts of each aspect of the Hope Model for each member: include a star for the goal, a stop sign for obstacles, and two large arrows
- Blank paper in folders, or notebooks, to serve as 'Hope Folders' for each group member
- Handouts of the Hope Model (Appendix N), one copy for each member
- Writing utensils
- Blank paper

Session Directions:

- Give a basic description of the 6-week hope group (duration and purpose).
- Ask each member what hope means to them. Ask them to include examples of hope in their lives, giving a few examples of what that looks like

(e.g., "hope is when I see someone stand up for a kid getting picked on after school").

- Distribute and describe the Hope Model handout (Appendix N). Note how everyone has goals in their lives (e.g., getting 100% on a spelling test), and everyone has obstacles that get in the way of goals (e.g., not finding time to study). People with hope use *pathways* thinking (thinking that identifies avenues/actions to get around obstacles), such as asking a parent to help with studying. Hopeful people also keep up their *willpower thinking* when they are not sure they can achieve a goal. Willpower thinking might include positive or motivational thoughts, such as, "I can get all the spelling words right," "I just need to study a little more," "I can ask for help," or "I know I can do it."
- Ask for a volunteer to hold up their handout (Appendix N) and practice explaining the Hope Model to the group, including an example from his/ her own life.
- Discuss why hope is important. Begin with asking members why it may be important for them to have hope in their lives. Ask them to work with a partner to write down words or phrases on a sheet of paper that describe some of the negative things (e.g. obstacles) that might be happening in their lives, or society.
- Ask each pair to share their brainstorm of concerns or obstacles that could be helped by hope. Discuss why they are important concerns to address.
- Hand a star cutout to each youth, asking them to write down one goal on their star. Ask each member to share their goal. Discuss whether each goal is realistic and achievable.
- Hand out a stop sign cutout to each member. Ask them to brainstorm possible obstacles they may experience in achieving their stated goal, then have them write those obstacles on the stop sign. Have them share, and note which they think is most likely to happen.
- Ask them to brainstorm examples of pathways around obstacles (remember, pathways are avenues/actions to get around obstacles).
- Hand out one arrow cutout to each member. Ask them to write down the pathways idea they liked the best. Then give them another arrow cutout and ask them to write down what they might say to themselves (e.g., willpower) to keep working toward the goal.
- Ask each member to stand up and demonstrate the entire Hope Model in relation to their goal, describing it as if they were telling a story (e.g., "My goal is to get better at playing basketball, but the obstacle is that I can't find a place to practice. A pathway I can use is to ask my sister to take me to a court on the weekends, because she has a car. My willpower thought is 'I'm going to keep practicing so I can get good at this'").

- Pass out and explain the Hope Folders: Members will use the folders to collect all their handouts and write comments on progress made toward goal achievement. Keep folders with you, handing them out to members to take home at the end of the six sessions.
- Ask members to write down one goal in their Hope Folder that they will work on over the next few weeks. It can be the one they just shared with the group or a new one. Ask them to share the goal, and brainstorm concrete steps for achieving it for that week.
- Process with the below questions.

Process Questions:

1. How do you define hope?
   ¿Cómo defines la palabra esperanza?

2. Does the Spanish-language word *'esperanza'* have a different meaning from the English word 'hope' that we've been talking about today, and if so, what is it?
   ¿Tiene la palabra esperanza un significado diferente de la palabra 'hope' en ingles de la cuál hemos estado hablando hoy, si lo tiene? ¿Cuál es?

3. How does it relate to what we've been talking about today?
   ¿Cómo se relaciona a lo que hemos estado hablando hoy?

4. Are there unique ways you as a Latino/a gain a sense of hope, or do you draw hope from unique role models or values related to being Latino/a?
   ¿Existen algunas maneras distintas en la cuál tú como Latino/a adquieres una noción de esperanza o existen algunas personas que te sirven como modelo a seguir en los valores de ser Latino/a?

5. What was it like to learn about hope today?
   ¿Qué te pareció el aprender sobre 'esperanza' en el día de hoy?

6. Is hope something you already think or know about in your life?
   ¿La esperanza es algo en lo que tú piensas o ya conoces en tu vida?

7. Why might hope be important for Latino/a youth in particular?
   ¿Por qué puede la esperanza ser importante para la juventud Latino/a an particular?

8. What was most important from group today that you want to take with you and use somehow?
   ¿Qué fue lo más importante de tu participación en el grupo de hoy que quieres llevar contigo y utilizar de alguna manera?

SESSION 2: HOPE TO TACKLE OBSTACLES

Session Goal: To identify solutions to life obstacles.

Time Needed: 35–40 minutes

Suggested Group Size: 2–15

Materials Needed:

- Create note cards with examples of hopeful/hopeless talk (Appendix O)
- Hope Folders
- Blank note cards, two per group member
- Writing utensils

Session Directions:

- Check in with members about progress toward their identified goals. Ask them to identify the next steps they plan to take to continue to work toward their goals.
- Ask members to name obstacles in their lives, drawing from the previous week's discussion. Use the below process questions as a guide.
- Discuss hopeful talk as one way to deal with obstacles. Hopeful talk includes phrases, sentences, or words we say or think to ourselves to help motivate us to get around obstacles and reach our goals. Describe the willpower piece of the Hope Model, which involves positive things you say to yourself to get around challenges and keep up hope.
- Ask members to discuss examples of hopeful and hopeless talk they have heard or used themselves. Discuss ways the talk affects them, and ways to protect themselves from it.
- Hand out two blank note cards to each member, asking members to write one hopeful and one hopeless statement that they have heard said about Latino/a teenagers.
- Combine members' responses with quotes from famous people (Appendix O).
- Ask members to take turns, picking a card and reading it aloud to the group. Ask them to categorize them into one of two groups—hopeful or hopeless (ideally taping them to one wall or placing them in two distinct piles in the center of the group's circle).
- Ask members to turn hopeless phrases into hopeful ones.
- Ask each to write one hopeful phrase that is meaningful to them in their folders. Ask them to share their favorite phrase.

Process Questions:

1. What are obstacles or challenges that Latino/a youth sometimes face?
   ¿Cuáles son los obstáculos o desafíos que a veces enfrenta la juventud Latino/a?

2. Do other groups face these obstacles?
   ¿Enfrentan otros grupos estos obstáculos?

3. Where do the obstacles that Latino/a youth face come from?
   ¿De dónde provienen los obstáculos que enfrenta la juventud Latino/a?

4. What are some of the strengths Latino/a youth have to help them combat obstacles?
   ¿Qué piensas tú ser la mayor capacidad que tiene la juventud Latino/a que los ayuda a combatir obstáculos?

5. How well do you feel you understand the differences between hopeful and hopeless statements?
   ¿Sientes que entiendes bien las diferencias entre las frases "tener esperanza" y "no tener esperanza"?

6. What have been the most difficult obstacles you have faced in your life?
   ¿Cuáles son los obstáculos más difíciles que has tenido que enfrentar en tu vida?

7. What have been the most important hopeful messages you have received in your life? From whom?
   ¿Cuáles son los mensajes más importantes de esperanza que has recibido en tu vida? ¿De quién provienen estos mensajes?

SESSION 3: HOPEFUL TALK: MAKING CARTOONS

Session Goals: To focus on hopeful talk, and identify pathways around obstacles.

Time Needed: 35–40 minutes

Suggested Group Size: 2–15

Materials Needed:

- Cartoon poster boards (an enlarged copy of the cartoon in Appendix P)
- Individual-sized cartoon handouts, one per member (Appendix P)
- Hope Folders
- Writing utensils

Session Directions:

- Welcome group and review Hope Model.
- Pass out Hope Folders, and check in with and process member's progress toward goals.
- Share and discuss what is happening in the cartoon poster (Appendix P), using the below process questions.
- Invite members to come up with a quote the boy might be saying in his thought bubble. Discuss why the boy might be thinking this thought.
- Pass out a handout of the cartoon (Appendix P) to each member, and ask them to write the words they choose for each of the thought bubbles of the cartoon.
- Have group members go around and share the words they wrote. Then, discuss other types of situations in which members find themselves facing obstacles.
- Invite members to draw their own cartoons on the blank cartoon pages (Appendix P). Have them share or act these out. Make sure they include some solutions to any challenges or obstacles.
- All handouts can be placed in the Hope Folder.

Process Questions:

1. Has something like the situation in the cartoon with the boy ever happened to you?
   ¿Te ha pasado algo igual a la experiencia que tuvo el niño en la caricatura?

2. How did you deal with it?
   ¿Cómo lo enfrentaste?

3. Which people (*family*, etc.) or things in your life help you?
   ¿Cuáles personas (familiares, etc.) o cosas te ayudan en tu vida?

4. What strengths from your culture help you address obstacles?
   ¿Qué puntos fuertes de tu cultura te ayudan a lidiar con los obstáculos?

5. Has there been a time you could not come up with a solution to a problem?
   ¿Ha habido alguna vez cuando no pudiste solucionar un problema?

6. Have you ever seen a friend or family member have trouble coming up with a solution to a problem?
   ¿Has visto alguna vez a un amigo o a un familiar tener dificultad en solucionar un problema?

7. What made it difficult for them?
   ¿Qué se le hizo difícil para ellos?

SESSION 4: MY HOPE CHEERING SECTION

Session Goal: To identify social supports, including family, in group members' lives.

Time Needed: 35–40 minutes

Suggested Group Size: 2–15

Materials Needed:

- A blank sheet of paper with the title My Hope Cheering Section at the top (Appendix Q)
- Hope Folders
- Writing utensils

Session Directions:

- Pass out Hope Folders, and check in with goal progress. Invite them to write on the goal page any successes, challenges, or new goals and actions to take. Share as a group.
- Explore who supports them, asking: Who do you trust to support you most? Why? How are they supportive? At what times do you need their support the most?
- Ask members to complete the Hope Cheering Section sheet by writing down people who are in their personal support group and who help them stay hopeful.
- Once the sheets are completed, designate three areas (e.g., corners) in the room: family, friends, and teachers/coaches. Ask any members who wrote down a family member (e.g., parent, *tio*, etc.) to stand in the family area. Repeat for the friends and teachers/coaches.
- Ask group members to come back to the circle and count how many names they wrote for family, friends, and for teachers/coaches. Ask them to move to the area of the room that represents the largest list they had, and to notice where people are standing.
- Ask members to identify additional persons or things in their cheering section that didn't fit under family, friends, and teachers/coaches.
- Add the Hope Cheering Section worksheet to the Hope Folders.

Process Questions:

1. What was it like to hear about other members' cheering sections?
   ¿Qué te pareció cuando oíste a otros miembros mencionar las personas que le dan ánimo?

2. What did you have in common and what was different?
   ¿Qué tuvieron en común y que diferencia tuvieron?

3. What surprised you about what others wrote in their cheering sections?
   ¿Qué te sorprendió sobre lo que otros escribieron en su hoja?

4. Why is having a cheering section important for facing obstacles and having hope?
   ¿Por qué es importante tener personas que nos den aliento para poder enfrentar nuestros obstáculos y tener esperanza?

5. Can you think of people in your school or life who need a larger cheering section? Why or why not?
   ¿Puedes pensar en alguien de tu escuela o en tu vida personal que necesite más personas que le den aliento? ¿Por qué si o por qué no?

6. What was most important about today that you want to take with you and use somehow?
   ¿Qué fue lo más importante sobre el día de hoy que quieres llevar contigo y poder utilizar de alguna manera?

SESSION 5: HOPEFUL REPORTING

Session Goal: To gain experience in narrating a hopeful story.

Time Needed: 35–40 minutes

Suggested Group Size: 2–15

Materials Needed:

- Hope Folders
- Blank paper
- Writing utensils (or members could use phones or other recorders, to record themselves)
- Tape recording of leader telling a hope story (see facilitator notes for an example)

Session Directions:

- Pass out Hope Folders, and check in and journal regarding goal progress.
- Remind them that next week is the final session.
- Explain that members will serve that day as 'reporters' for one another. They are going to interview one other person in the group about their goal, and then share with the rest of the group that person's unique hope story. A person's hope story can be the goal the member has been working on, or some other goal. As part of their reporting, members should ask additional questions to get details so they can make the story interesting.
- Play the recording of the group leader telling a hope story.
- Give every member a piece of paper and writing utensils (or recorder) and divide the group into pairs. Designate who are the reporters and who are the interviewees for the first round.
- Give members 5 minutes to be interviewed.
- After 5 minutes, ask group members to switch roles and repeat the process.
- Once finished, put members' names in a pile and draw a person's name who will 'report' his interview to the entire group. If time permits, pick additional members' names.

Process Questions:

1. What was it like to interview your friend?
   ¿Qué te pareció al entrevistar a tu amigo?

2. What did you learn that was new about your friend?
    ¿Aprendiste algo nuevo que no sabías sobre tu amigo?

3. What is it like to tell a hope story?
    ¿Qué te pareció al relatar una historia de esperanza?

4. What are the challenges you encountered in telling an interesting story?
    ¿Encontraste alguna dificultad en relatar una historia interesante?

5. What themes did you notice that were similar across the stories you heard?
    ¿De las historias que escuchaste hubieron temas similares?

6. What is most meaningful that you heard or did today that you will take with you?
    ¿Qué fue lo más importante que oíste o hiciste en el día de hoy que llevarás contigo?

Facilitator Notes: Example of interview: Good afternoon. We are reporting from Hope High School and I am talking with Mr. Dave. Mr. Dave has been working hard at getting along with his brother over the past weeks. They seem to fight a lot but he has been trying to find ways to get along. When his brother comes into his room when he's doing homework, Mr. Dave has stopped yelling at him and instead asks him nicely to leave. If his brother doesn't leave, Mr. Dave picks up his stuff and goes to another room in the house. So far this has worked twice, but Mr. Dave will see if it continues. Stay tuned for what will happen next . . .

SESSION 6: HOPE FOR THE FUTURE

Session Goal: To apply the Hope Model to group members' lives by creating a hope collage.

Time needed: 35–40 minutes

Suggested Group Size: 2–15

Materials Needed:

- Scissors
- Hope Folders
- Glue/glue sticks
- Large construction paper
- Magazines or cut out pictures with images of people, places, or objects
- Markers/colored pencils/crayons

Session Directions:

- Discuss final progress made on personal goals, their various experiences attempting to achieve their goals, and what they have learned about goal achievement across the sessions. Also discuss any remaining steps they have to reach their goals.
- Explain that today they are going create 'hope collages' that show what hope means to each person. Members can draw or cut out pictures or write words—however they want to fill their page. They can also include the goal they have been working on.
- Give each member a piece of construction paper and lay out the magazines for all to use in creating their individual collage.
- After approximately 15 minutes, ask each member to share their collage with the group. After each member shares, ask the others to state one strength they have seen in this peer over the course of the group which they believe will help him/her remain hopeful in the future.
- Give group members their Hope Folders to take home.

Process Questions:

1. What did you learn from this group?
   ¿Qué aprendiste de este grupo?

2. What was it like being in the group?
   ¿Cómo te sentiste al pertenecer a este grupo?

3. What session or activity did you like best in this group, and why?
   ¿Qué parte o actividad disfrutaste más de este grupo? Explica.

4. Which session or activity did you like least, and why?
   ¿Qué parte o actividad fue la que menos te gustó de este grupo? Explica.

5. How has what you learned during group helped you?
   ¿Cómo te ha ayudado lo que aprendiste durante tu participación en grupo?

6. How can you share hope with other people in your life or community?
   ¿Cómo puedes dar experanza a otras personas en tu vida o en tu comunidad?

REFERENCES

Edwards, L. M., & Lopez, S. J. (2000). *Making hope happen for kids*. Unpublished protocol. University of Kansas, Lawrence.

Pedrotti, J. T., Lopez, S. J., & Krieshok, T. (2000). *Making hope happen: A program for fostering strengths in adolescents*. Unpublished protocol. University of Kansas, Lawrence.

The Hope Model

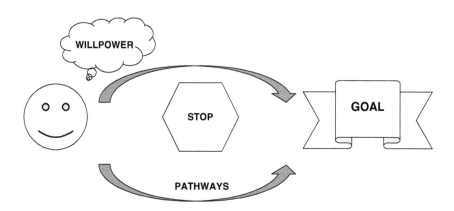

Hope is made of goals, pathways, and willpower. Imagine that you are the smiley face, and you have a goal you are working toward. You will always have obstacles (the stop sign) that get in the way of your goals. To get around the stop sign, you will need to use pathways thinking to come up with alternative routes around the obstacles. You will also need to use willpower thinking to keep yourself motivated and positive. With these two types of thinking, you will be able to make progress toward your goals and have hope for the future!

Figure 7.1   The Hope Model

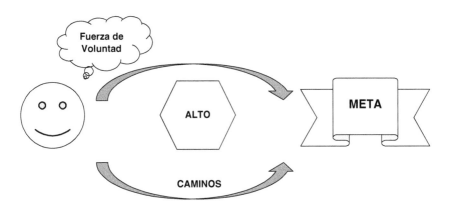

La esperanza está compuesta de metas, caminos, y fuerza de voluntad. Imagina que eres la carita sonriente y que te has trazado una meta. Con frecuencia tendrás obstáculos (la señal de ALTO) que estorbará el camino a tu meta. Para combatir la señal de alto, tendrás que imaginarte una trayectoria diferente para combatir los obstáculos. También tendrás que tener fuerza de voluntad para mantenerte motivado y positivo. Con estos dos modelos diferentes de pensar serás capaz de alcanzar tus metas y tener esperanza en el futuro.

Figure 7.2   Modelo de Esperanza

Hopeful/Hopeless Talk Examples

HOPEFUL TALK EXAMPLES

1. "If you're trying to achieve, there will be roadblocks. I've had them, everybody has had them. But obstacles don't have to stop you. If you run into a wall, don't turn around and give up. Figure out how to climb it, go through it, or work around it." (Michael Jordan, well-known basketball player)
   "Si tratas de alcanzar algo vas a tener estorbos. Yo los he tenido, todos los hemos tenido. Pero los obstáculos no deben detenerte. Si encuentras una pared, no te des por vencido. Figúrate como puedes subirla, penetrarla, o ir alrededor de ella."(Michael Jordan, un jugador de baloncesto muy conocido)

2. "Si se puede!"/"Yes, it can be done!" (Cesar Chavez, an American farm worker, labor leader, and civil rights activist who, with Dolores Huerta, co-founded the National Farm Workers Association. A Mexican American, Chavez became the best-known Latino/a American civil rights activist)
   "¡Si se puede!"(César Chávez, un campesino mexicoestadounidense, líder y activista por los derechos civiles, junto a Dolores Huerta, fundó la Asociación Nacional de Agricultores)

3. "I've only scratched the surface of where I want to be in my career . . . And I know one thing, I haven't won anything yet so there's a lot more I can do there. But I'm going to continue to get better and do what I can to help my team be the best it can possibly be." (Dwayne Wade, a Miami Heat basketball player)
   "Yo solo he rascado la superficie de a donde quiero llegar en my profesión . . . Y sé una cosa, no he ganado nada todavía, lo que significa que aún tengo más que hacer. Pero voy a continuar mejorando para que mi equipo sea lo mejor que puede ser." (Dwayne Wade, jugador de baloncesto del equipo Miami Heat)

HOPELESS TALK EXAMPLES

1. "I really like playing basketball, but I am the shortest one in class. I will never be any good."
   "Me gusta mucho jugar baloncesto, pero soy el más bajo de la clase. Nunca seré un buen jugador."

2. "School is hard. Just when I think my grades are going up I fail a quiz. Sometimes I get so frustrated."

"La escuela se me hace muy difícil. Cada vez que creo que voy bien, me va mal en un examen. A veces me siento frustrado/a."

3. "My brothers and sisters drive me crazy. I don't know how I can live in the same house with them."
"Mis hermanos y mis hermanas me vuelven loco. No se como puedo vivir en la misma casa con ellos."

Cartoon Handouts

Hoja de Caricaturas

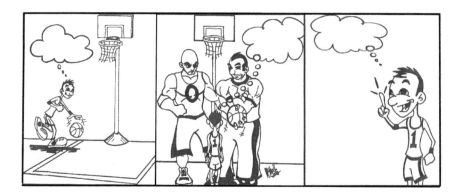

Figure 7.3   Cartoon Poster Board

Figure 7.4   Hopeful Cartoons

My Hope Cheering Section

Lo que me da Ánimo

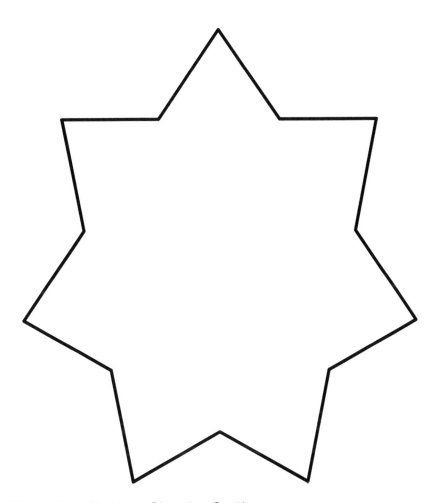

Figure 7.5   My Hope Cheering Section

LATINO/A YOUTH AND HEALTHY RELATIONSHIPS

José M. Maldonado and Pietro Sasso

SESSION 1: COMMUNICATION AND FAMILY RELATIONSHIPS

Session Goal: To foster awareness regarding communication and relationship styles.

Time Needed: 30–45 minutes

Suggested Group Size: 2–15

Materials Needed:

- One genogram cheat sheet (Appendix R) per group member, extras in case of mistakes
- The facilitator's own family genogram, as an example
- Writing utensils
- Markers/colored pencils/crayons

Session Directions:

- Define open and closed communication (see definitions below, under facilitator notes). Give examples that match the developmental level and context of group members.
- Provide an explanation of the family genogram, using the facilitator's genogram as an example. Share something personal (such as a family

pattern of conflict between men in the family), to role model a deeper level of genogram construction and discussion.

- Hand out a genogram cheat sheet page (Appendix R) to each member, asking them to create their genogram, with directions as follows:

  ▢ Write family names representing each family member onto the genogram, adding additional members beyond the current family symbols provided on the sheet. Stress that family can be anyone who has been very important to their development, giving examples: birth parents, grandparents, *padrinos* (godparents), foster parents, adoptive parents, aunts, uncles, cousins, neighbors, etc.

  ▢ If they wish, members can draw an 'x' through deceased family members or, conversely, create their own mark to indicate deceased.

  ▢ Indicate the type of relationship between members: Ask them to draw a solid, connecting line between family members who are very close or who have positive relationships. Draw a jagged line (like a lightning bolt) between family members who are in conflict or who are disconnected.

- Ask members to indicate communication styles used in their families (open versus closed, or a bit of both). Stress that communication styles may differ between people or according to topics (e.g., most families are closed on topics related to sex and politics).

  ▢ Ask them to draw an 'O' to indicate open, and a 'C' to indicate closed, regarding communication styles. This can be drawn at the top of the paper, if the family overall has one style, or can be placed next to certain members to indicate different family members with different styles.

  ▢ For those who indicated 'closed' on their sheet, have them list all the topics that are hidden/closed and for whom (give examples: e.g., kids not allowed to discuss topics such as sex or religion; men not allowed to reveal certain emotions).

- Once complete, each member shares with the entire group, as comfortable.
- Facilitate a discussion with the below questions.

Process Questions

1. What emotions or feelings did you experience as you created your genogram? *¿Cuáles emociones sentiste cuando hiciste el genograma?*

2. What patterns (Conflicts? Open or closed communication styles? Or losses?) did you notice across your family, and how do you feel about them?

¿Cuáles conflictos, estilo de comunicación abierta o cerrada, o pérdidas notaste en tu familia y que piensas sobre esto?

3. Talk about how certain patterns are related to your Latino/a heritage; which are related to gender roles and norms?
   Habla sobre como ciertos modelos están relacionados a tu herencia Latina, ¿y cuáles están relacionados a las normas y roles de género?

4. What was it like hearing about others' families and their communication styles?
   ¿Qué te pareció al darte cuenta de los estilos de comunicación que existen en otras familias?

5. What did you notice about what topics tend to be 'closed/taboo' in families?
   ¿Qué notaste sobre los temas que tienden ser 'cerrados/prohibidos' en las familias?

6. Is the open or closed communication style better? What do you think is 'most healthy'?
   ¿Cuál estilo de comunicación es mejor, abierto o cerrado? ¿Cuál de los dos piensas es el más saludable?

7. How do you feel about the communication between you and your family?
   ¿Cómo te sientes sobre el estilo de comunicación que tienes con tu familia?

8. In what ways would you like to improve certain patterns in your family—and what are you doing to change it, in your own relationships?
   ¿En qué manera te gustaría mejorar ciertas cosas en tu familia—y qué estás haciendo para cambiarlas en tus propias relaciones?

Facilitator Notes: The facilitator should be aware of possible emotional reactions to constructing genograms, as they can elicit painful memories/reactions that may be inappropriate to address in that setting. Stress that the setting and limited time frame do not allow for in-depth storytelling, nor the telling of personal events that will make them uncomfortable.

Open Communication: Family members communicate and foster open discussions about most topics, experiences, mental health issues, or emotions (Shearman & Dumlao, 2008). Closed Communication: A system of communication where discussing many 'sensitive' topics, experiences, mental health issues, or emotions is taboo/not allowed, emphasizing instead the need to uphold a shared value or belief system rather than individual expressions. Closed communication may lead to indirect communication styles and family secrets (adapted from Shearman & Dumlao, 2008).

SESSION 2: SINGING THE LANGUAGE OF RELATIONSHIPS

Session Goal: To facilitate group members' expression of relationships through song.

Time Needed: 30–45 minutes

Suggested Group Size: 2–15

Materials Needed:

- Multiple recordings of song selections (or copies of song lyrics) that emphasize relationships with friends, adults, family members, and extended family
- Ahead of time, such as in the first session, members can be encouraged to reflect on songs that talk about relationships
- Paper
- Writing utensils

Session Directions:

- Explain how musical expression can communicate ideas about healthy/ unhealthy relationships, values, and/or stories. As an example, select and play a song that reflects relationship themes, cultural communication, and significant values.
- Ask group members to brainstorm songs that convey various forms of relationships.
- Several members can share their relationship songs by singing or playing the song, with a time limit for each musical expression of 2–3 minutes.
- After members finish sharing, process with the below questions, with efforts to highlight cultural themes that influence positive aspects of relationships and good communication.
- If there is time, ask members to construct, in groups or alone, their own songs or poems about relationships, or hopes for future relationships.

Process Questions:

1. What song most expressed your perceptions of healthy relationships, and how so?
   ¿Cuál canción expresó tu percepción sobre una relación saludable, y cómo lo expresó?

2. How does music help you express your feelings about relationships?
   ¿Cómo te ayuda la música a expresar tus emociones sobre las relaciones?

3. If your song was negative in some way (such as lyrics promoting violence or drug use), how can you use it to create good and positive things in your life?

   Si tu canción mostró negatividad de alguna manera (si las letras promueven la violencia o el uso de las drogas), ¿Cómo la puedes usar para crear algo positivo en tu vida?

4. What did you learn, hearing others discuss healthy and unhealthy relationships?

   ¿Qué aprendiste al escuchar a otros discutir el tema de relaciones saludables y no saludables?

5. Is there music that better reflects your own cultural beliefs about relationships? Which? How so?

   ¿Existe alguna música que refleje tus propias creencias culturales sobre las relaciones? ¿Cuál es? ¿Cómo lo refleja?

6. What does the activity tell you overall about yourself? Others?

   ¿Qué te dice esta actividad en general sobre ti? ¿Sobre otros?

7. What was most meaningful about writing your own, or hearing others', songs?

   ¿Qué fue lo más significativo sobre escribir tus propias canciones o escuchar las canciones de otros?

SESSION 3: LET'S MOTIVATE OURSELVES: FINDING THE LEADER WITHIN!

Session Goal: Group members identify leadership qualities in themselves and others.

Time Needed: 30–45 minutes

Suggested Group Size: 2–15

Materials Needed:

- A variety of age-appropriate magazines
- Newspapers
- Scissors
- Tape/glue
- Blank paper
- Markers/colored pencils/crayons
- Poster board for the facilitator to write on

Session Directions:

- Brainstorm positive leaders in their lives. Ask them to explain what makes them positive, as well as 'leaders.'
- Ask them to identify leadership qualities of those leaders, while you write them on the board, such as: Integrity, resiliency/ability to overcome difficulties, ability to inspire/motivate others, humility, effective communication skills (such as clear communication, assertiveness, and optimism/positivity), openness to new ideas, creativity. Additional leadership skills emphasized with children and youth are charisma, curiosity, adventure, and inspiration.
- Asking members to keep these qualities in mind, have members create a collage of what they see as the most important leadership qualities they would like to possess.
- Have them share their collages. Discuss ways they can gain preferred leadership qualities.
- If members know each other well enough: Ask them to turn over their collages and go around and write on others' papers one leadership quality they see in the other. After, ask them to silently read what peers wrote about them, and discuss their reactions.

Process Questions:

1. In picking your leader, what about him/her was most important to you?
   ¿Cuándo escogiste a tu líder, que fue lo más importante para ti sobre él?

2. What leadership traits do you share with your leader?
   ¿Cuáles rasgos de liderazgo compartes con tu líder?

3. What was it like to read what your peers thought about your leadership qualities?
   ¿Qué te pareció al leer lo que pensaron tus compañeros de tus cualidades de liderazgo?

4. Were they right? Did they miss any?
   ¿Estaban en lo correcto o pasaron por alto algunas cualidades?

5. Which leadership traits do you want to develop, and how will you develop those?
   ¿Cuáles cualidades de liderazgo quieres desarrollar y como lo harías?

6. How might you use such traits in your future?
   ¿Cómo utilizarías estas cualidades en tu futuro?

7. How can they help you in your future career?
   ¿Cómo te pueden ayudar en tu carrera futura?

8. What is one thing you'll do this week, to use or develop one leadership quality?
   ¿Cuál sería una cosa que vas hacer esta semana para usar o desarrollar una cualidad de liderazgo?

SESSION 4: LOST IN TRANSLATION: HURTFUL LANGUAGE

Session Goal: Identify and practice respectful forms of communication.

Time Needed: 30–45 minutes

Suggested Group Size: 2–15

Materials Needed:

■ Index cards
■ Writing utensils
■ Copies of Bias Language handout (Appendix S), one for each group member
■ One shoebox with a slit several inches wide cut into the lid

Session Directions:

■ Explain that you will review biased terms and statements that can 'hurt' others, exploring what about them may hurt, while creating healthier ways to communicate.
■ Distribute Bias Language handout (Appendix S) to each group member and ask them to take turns reading biased terms out loud, in both English and Spanish.
■ After, explore youth reactions to the statements, asking group members to address in their dyad the following questions:

❑ What are your reactions to the language or statements we just read?
¿Cuál es tu reacción con referencia al lenguaje o frases que acabamos de leer?

❑ These terms were identified as biased—what does 'biased' mean?
Estás palabras se identifican con ser prejuiciosas—¿Qué significa la palabra 'prejuicio'?

❑ What about the language might be biased?
¿Cómo puede ser el lenguaje prejuicioso?

❑ How might the language/terms hurt or offend some?
¿Cómo pueden estas palabras ofender a alguien?

❑ What bugs you, and why?
¿Qué te molesta, y por qué?

■ Have group members share their conclusions as an entire group.
■ Hand out several index cards to the dyads, asking members to work in their dyad to generate and write down additional 'biased language/

phrases' that they hear all around them, such as words or phrases that can be perceived as offensive, racist, or sexist.

- While they are doing this, the facilitator could write several on index cards and put them in the shoebox.
- Have group members insert their cards into the shoebox.
- Shake the shoebox and assign an equal amount of index cards to each dyad.
- Ask them to brainstorm in the dyad ways to change words or phrases to make them more respectful. Ask them to write the new word or phrase on the other side of the index card.
- Have the dyads put all the index cards into the shoebox, then ask members to randomly pull cards from the shoebox, one at a time, to read and identify with peers the offensive/disrespectful statements and the suggested solutions.
- Ask them to discuss their opinions of each card, such as whether they believe the suggested new language is respectful or if there are kinder words.
- Ask members to practice a role play, whereby they confront a peer who is using language that offends them or that is biased (you can also pick biased/offensive language used commonly in your setting). Make sure to switch roles, so that every person gets a chance to role play both roles. You can also offer a role play that models effective (e.g., positive, non-violent) confrontation.
- Process afterward, to explore what is difficult about confronting others.

Process Questions:

1. How do words show our biases about certain groups?
   ¿Cómo muestran las palabras nuestros prejuicios hacia ciertos grupos?

2. How might language affect how you see others?
   ¿Cómo puede el lenguaje afectar como percibes a otras personas?

3. Where do we learn those biases/beliefs?
   ¿De dónde aprendemos esos prejuicios o creencias?

4. How do those words hurt others? Ourselves? Do words cause violence against groups?
   ¿Cómo pueden esas palabras lastimar a otros? ¿A nosotros mismos? ¿Causan violencia estas palabras hacia ciertos grupos?

5. How might we bully with words? How do we use social media to bully?
   ¿Cómo podemos intimidar a otras personas con nuestras palabras? ¿Cómo usamos los medios de comunicación para intimidar?

6. What are the differences in the new words or phrases used that you suggested?
   ¿Cuáles son las diferencias en las palabras o frases nuevas que sugeriste?

7. Was it difficult making words more respectful?
   ¿Fue difícil cambiar las palabras para hacerlas más respetuosas?

8. Will you use these new, more respectful words outside of this room, and where/with whom?
   ¿Vas a utilizar estas nuevas palabras, las cuales son más respetuosas, fuera de esta sala, con quién y en dónde?

SESSION 5: MALE/FEMALE GENDER ROLE BOX

Session Goal: To identify healthy and unhealthy gender roles, stereotypes, expectations.

Time Needed: 30–45 minutes

Suggested Group Size: 2–15

Materials Needed:

- Poster paper or board
- Markers/colored pencils/crayons
- Writing utensils
- Blank paper

Session Directions:

- Draw a large box on the board or poster paper, with sufficient room to write both in and around the box.
- Ask members if they have ever heard someone being told to "act like a man," "be macho," or "man up." Encourage a discussion on the topic and share an example, to help members conceptualize the idea. On the contrary, ask members if they have ever heard someone being told to "act like a lady," "be a lady," or "be lady-like."
- After the discussion, write "Act like a Man" on the top of the box. Ask members to shout out what this means in their community, family, and to them. Then write "Act like a Lady" on the top of the box, asking members to shout out what it means in their community to 'act like a lady'—what are the expectations as they perceive them?
- Invite group members to write in the box words they think describe what it means to act like a man or act like a lady. Prompts may include how a 'real man' expresses feelings (love, sadness, hurt), how they are supposed to treat women, how Latino men act, etc. They may also include how a girl/lady expresses feelings (love, sadness, hurt), how Latinas are supposed to treat men, how Latina women act, how to be feminine, how women deal with conflict.
- After the box is filled, process responses. Address traditional roles, stereotypes, unrealistic expectations, positive and negative roles, and cultural influences.
- Ask the question, are men/women stuck inside this box? If yes, which men/women? And who forces them to stay there?

- Invite members to circle roles etc. in the box they would like to change.
- State the group is now going to move "outside the box," asking them to describe behaviors of boys or men and girls or women that are outside the box in some way (actions/ways of being that are more realistic/real or human). Give an example or use the circled words to ask them to think of alternatives. Write examples outside and around the box.
- Hand out paper to each and various colored pens/markers. Ask group members to "open their boxes" and create a new vision of what they think men, women, boys, and girls should be like.

  ❏ Ask them to include how they want to change, and ways to make this happen. Give them time; encourage creativity and use of words, phrases, drawings.

- Ask group members to share their visions, or to at least name what they plan to do differently, to "open up their boxes."

Process Questions:

1. What words outside of the box are positive to you?
   ¿Cuáles palabras fuera del cuadro son positivas para ti?

2. What words outside of the box are negative/bad to you or others?
   ¿Cuáles palabras fuera del cuadro son negativas para ti o para otros?

3. What do we learn about these things outside this box? Is it positive, negative; how so?
   ¿Qué aprendemos de las cosas fuera del cuadro? ¿Son positivas o negativas? ¿Cómo lo son?

4. What happens when guys act outside the box? How might this lead to bullying, and have you ever noticed that in your schools, families, or neighborhoods?
   ¿Qué pasa cuando los hombres actúan fuera del cuadro? ¿Cómo puede esto llevar a la intimidación, y has visto esto en tu escuela, en tu familia, o en tu vecindario?

5. How do you treat guys who are outside the box?
   ¿Cómo tratas a los hombres que están fuera del cuadro?

6. What might change in all of our lives, for both guys and girls, if we let men and boys be more outside the box?
   ¿Qué cambiaría en nuestras vidas, para ambos hombres y mujeres, si permitiéramos que los hombres y los niños vivan fuera del cuadro?

7. Is there a way to be 'macho' that could be positive and loving?
   ¿Existe una manera de ser 'macho' que puede ser positiva y amorosa?

8. How can we begin to open the box, to let men and boys be more 'real' and human—and do we want to? If yes, what can we begin to do differently?
   ¿Cómo podemos empezar a abrir el cuadro para dejar que los hombres y los niños sean más 'reales' y humanos—o queremos que esto ocurra? Si la respuesta es sí, ¿Podemos hacer algo diferente?

Facilitator Notes: This exact session can be done with a focus on females and their expected gender roles.

SESSION 6: HOW TO 'FIGHT FAIR' IN RELATIONSHIPS

Session Goal: To learn healthy conflict resolution skills.

Time Needed: 30–45 minutes

Suggested Group Size: 5–15

Materials Needed:

- Large poster board
- Writing utensils
- Index cards
- Box
- Fighting Fair handout (Appendix T)

Session Directions:

- Ask members to define the term 'relationship,' and to note strengths of their relationships.
- Note that all relationships have disagreements. Ask them to identify what they most disagree, fight, or argue about in their relationships.
- Explain that there are ways to 'fight fair' that can actually improve relationships. Ask them to list both good and bad ways to fight. If some suggestions are negative (such as 'punch' or 'call names'), ask others if they agree and encourage debate.
- Ask if there are any gender or cultural expectations or norms for ways to communicate or behave in their relationships.
- Have members write their responses on the poster board, and process.
- Hand out the Fighting Fair handout (Appendix T). Process the handout and how easy or difficult it may be to adhere to such ideas.
- Provide a scenario of an argument/disagreement that is common to the group members' age or context (or ask them to provide one).
- Hand out index cards. Have members use the fighting fair list to develop a healthy way to work out the scenario. Have them write ideas down on an index card.
- After each scenario, have members put all responses in a box. The facilitator can pull out and share responses, asking members to discuss which are best, and why. Potentially have members role play a best solution.

Process Questions:

1. What was the most important thing we talked about today?
    ¿Qué fue lo más importante de lo que hablamos hoy?

2. What did you learn about fighting fair?
    ¿Qué aprendiste sobre la lucha justa?

3. What new skill do you want to take with you and try this week?
    ¿Qué quieres llevarte contigo y hacer esta semana?

4. With whom will you try it out?
    ¿Con quién lo vas a tratar?

5. What might prevent you from actually changing your ways?
    ¿Qué puede impedir en que cambies tu manera de pelear/discutir?

6. How can we give support to help you change some style of fighting that you want to change?
    ¿Cómo podemos darte apoyo para ayudarte a cambiar el estilo de pelear que tú quieres cambiar?

REFERENCES

Gottman, J. M., & Silver, N. (2000). *The 7 principles for making marriage work.* New York, NY: Three Rivers Press

Shearman, S. M., & Dumlao, R. (2008). A cross-cultural comparison of family communication patterns and conflict between young adults and parents. *Journal of Family Communication, 8*(3), 186–211. doi:10.1080/15267430802182456

Genogram Example

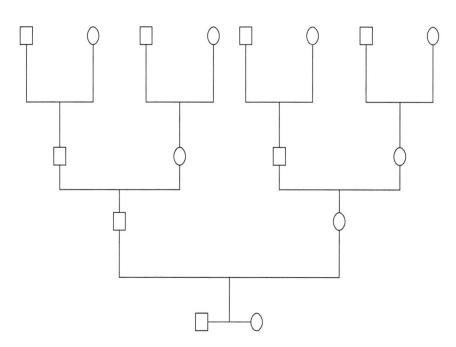

Figure 8.1   Genogram Example

Bias Language Handout

Workman's compensation (*compensación laboral*)
Woman's intuition (*intuición de mujer*)
Mankind (*humanidad/género humano*)
Manmade (*hecho por el hombre*)
Old wives' tale (*cuento de vieja*)
Sportsmanship (*espíritu deportivo*)
Cleaning lady (*señora de la limpieza*)
Freshman (*Estudiante de primer ano*)
Man and wife (*hombre y mujer*)
You guys (*ustedes/vosotros*)
Bachelor's degree (*Bachiller*)
Stewardess (*azafata*)
Machismo (*machismo*)
White lie (*mentira piadosa*)
Layman (*lego*)
Tomboy (*marimacho*)
Policeman (*policía*)
Manhole (*pozo*)
Housewife (*ama de casa*)
Congressman (*congresista*)
Landlord (*propietario*)
Black lie (*mentira negra*)
Waitress (*mesera*)
Macho (*macho*)
Male nurse (*enfermero*)
Illegal alien (*inmigrante ilegal*)
Minority (*minoría*)
Chairman (*presidente*)
Black hole (*calabozo*)

Rules for Fair Fights

*Adapted from Gottman, 2000

Start kind: When you first speak, try to say something positive first. If you are angry at your mom, start with a "Hello" (and maybe even a "how was your day?") before you ask her to listen to your complaint.

Escucha a la otra persona: Escuchar es también algo muy difícil de hacer—intenta sentarte en silencio y escuchar lo que dice la otra persona y oblígate a NO pensar sobre lo que vas a responder.

Start with "I": Use "I" language. "I was mad that you grounded me" sounds better than "You always ground me for nothing."

Empieza con "Yo": Incluye la palabra "yo." "Yo estaba enfadado porque me castigaste," suena mejor que "Tú siempre me castigas por nada."

Accept responsibility: Be honest about your role in the situation. "I know I came home late. But I'm still angry that you grounded me for a whole month . . . " This is much better than "I didn't do anything wrong and you grounded me for a whole month!"

Acepta responsabilidad: Sé honesto sobre tu rol en la situación. "Yo sé que llegué tarde a casa. Pero todavia estoy enfadado porque me castigó durante todo un mes . . . " Esto es mucho mejor que "¡Yo no hice nada malo y me castigó durante todo un mes!"

Admit when you are wrong!: This is very hard and brave to do.

¡Admite cuando estés equivocado!: Esto es muy difícil y valiente de hacer.

Listen to the other person: Listening is also very hard to do—try sitting in silence and hearing what someone else says, and force yourself NOT to think about what you are going to say in response.

Escucha a la otra persona: Escuchar es también algo muy difícil de hacer—intenta sentarte en silencio y escuchar a lo que dice otra persona y obligáte a NO pensar sobre lo que vas a responder.

After listening, show that you heard: Repeat what the other person said, to show you heard correctly: Instead of firing back an insult or defense, repeat what he/she said. This DOES NOT mean you are agreeing. Example: "So you're mad that I ignored you all night at the party and you feel like I do this at every party we go to?"

Después de escuchar, muestra que escuchaste: Repite lo que dijo la otra persona, para mostrar que escuchaste correctamente: En vez de disparar un insulto o defensa, repite lo que él/ella dijo. Esto NO significa que tú estás en acuerdo. Por ejemplo: "Estás enojado porque yo te ignoré toda la noche en la fiesta y sientes que yo hago esto en cada fiesta que asistimos."

Tell the other person/be honest: If it is safe to do so, tell the other person the truth if something they did/said hurt you. Ask them to stop this behavior and explain that you can no longer be friends if they continue to treat you badly.
Pídele a la otra persona que sea honesta: *Si es seguro hacerlo, dile la verdad si algo que ellos dijeron o hicieron te hirió. Pídele que paren ese comportamiento y explícales que tú ya no deseas mantener su amistad si ellos continúan tratándote mal.*

Use kind language (e.g., words do hurt, people never forget them!): No name calling, sarcasm, contempt (e.g., tearing someone apart/criticizing them), bringing up the past, or being cruel. This destroys relationships over time.
Usa lenguaje amable (p. ej., ¡Las palabras duelen, la gente nunca las olvida¡): *No insultos, sarcasmo, o desprecio (p. ej. criticar a alguien), traer cosas del pasado, o ser cruel. A medida que pasa el tiempo esto destruye las relaciones.*

If you can't be kind, walk away: Come back when you're cooler, or write a letter. But if you always walk away and never try to work it out, this also kills a relationship.
Si no puedes ser amable, sigue tu camino: *Regresa cuando estés más calmado, o escribe una carta. Pero si siempre evitas la situación y no tratas de resolverla, esto también acaba con una relación.*

Compromise: Find a creative way to get you AND the other person's needs met. For instance, "I know you don't want me to go to parties with friends, but friends are important to me. How about I go to parties where you can call the parents, to talk to them to make sure they'll be there?"
Compromiso: *Encuentra una manera creativa para responder a tus necesidades Y las necesidades de otras personas. Por ejemplo, "Yo se que tú no quieres que yo vaya a las fiestas con mis amigos, pero los amigos son importantes para mi. ¿Por qué no voy a fiestas dónde puedas llamar a los padres y hablar con ellos para asegurarte que ellos estarán ahí?"*

Ask for a specific, concrete solution, and listen to his/her ideas too: Instead of, "I'll just help around the house some time . . . " specifically say, "I'll do the laundry once a week, and mow the lawn too."
Pide soluciones concretas y específicas, y también escucha sus ideas: *En vez de, "Yo a veces ayudaré en la casa . . . "di específicamente, "Yo lavaré la ropa una vez por semana y también cortaré el césped."*

PROMOTING CRITICAL CONSCIOUSNESS IN LATINO/A YOUTH

Ijeoma Ezeofor, Jamie C. Welch, and Richard Q. Shin

SESSION 1: OUR SOCIAL IDENTITIES

Session Goal: To explore social identities.

Time Needed: 30–45 minutes

Suggested Group Size: 2–15

Materials Needed:

- Two pieces of blank paper for each member
- Writing utensils

Session Directions:

- Ask participants for their definition of diversity. Generally, you are looking for answers that acknowledge the great diversity both across individuals and within social groups (e.g., Latinos, Catholics, etc.).
- Hand out one sheet of paper and ask members to write down the following (or create a handout with these categories on them): name and nickname; three words that describe yourself; favorite (movie, hobby, book,

song, artist, food, etc.); personal motto; greatest hero; strength; skill of which you are proud.

■ Ask members to share responses with the group.

■ Ask them to explore additional ways people differ, focusing on social identities (e.g., race, sexual orientation, gender identity). Supplement with some definitions (Appendix U). Ask them to consider: religion, race, socioeconomic status, abilities (physical, emotional, developmental), sexual orientation, sex, gender role.

■ Give members the other sheet of paper and ask them to define and write examples of their personal social identities.

■ Have members share their identities in a dyad, then with the entire group, as comfortable.

■ Ask which identity is most important or meaningful to them, and why.

Process Questions:

1. What was it like to share your identities?
   ¿Cómo fue el compartir tus identidades?

2. Where do we learn our social identities? Do they change?
   ¿De dónde aprendemos nuestras identidades sociales? ¿Estas identidades cambian?

3. Are all social identities treated the same?
   ¿Son todas las identidades sociales tratadas de la misma manera?

4. Do you have any identities that are stigmatized/discriminated against? Does this make it more difficult to talk about them?
   ¿Tienes identidades que son estigmatizadas o discriminadas? ¿Hace esto que sea más difícil de hablar de ellas?

5. What was most important about today's discussion that you want to remember?
   ¿Qué fue lo más importante sobre la discusión de hoy que quieres llevar contigo?

6. How did this activity deal with social justice?
   ¿Cómo trató esta actividad el tema de la justicia social?

Facilitator Notes: Have members give their identity descriptors to you, to bring back weekly.

SESSION 2: EXPLORING PRIDE AND RESILIENCY

Session Goal: To identify sources of pride and resiliency related to personal identities.

Time Needed: 20–30 minutes

Suggested Group Size: 2–15

Materials Needed:

- Coat of Arms handout (Appendix V), one for each member
- Markers/colored pencils/crayons
- Writing utensils

Session Directions:

- Have each member fill out a Coat of Arms (Appendix V), writing their names on the side with six quadrants, and writing or drawing answers to the questions in each quadrant.
- After they are completed, have group members share in dyads and then the larger group.
- Collect shields at the end, noting that you will bring them back to subsequent sessions, to provide a sense of strength and comfort to members as they discuss emotionally provocative issues in the sessions to come.

Process Questions:

1. What was most important about your answers?
   ¿De tus respuestas, qué fue lo más importante?

2. Does your shield look like anyone else's?
   ¿Se parece tu escudo al de otra persona?

3. How is it different?
   ¿Cómo es diferente?

4. Why is it different?
   ¿Por qué es diferente?

5. How did you feel while doing this activity?
   ¿Cómo te sentiste mientras hacías esta actividad?

6. What did you learn about yourself?
   ¿Qué aprendiste sobre ti?

7. About others?
   ¿Qué aprediste sobre otras personas?

8. What is most meaningful about today's group that you will remember?
   ¿Qué es lo más significativo del día de hoy sobre el grupo que vas a recordar?

SESSION 3: LEARNING ABOUT DISCRIMINATION, OPPRESSION, AND PRIVILEGE

Session Goal: To learn how discrimination, oppression, and privilege affect them and others.

Time Needed: 30–45 minutes

Suggested Group Size: 2–15

Materials Needed:

- 'D-O-P' vignettes (Appendix W)

Session Directions:

- Ask group members split up into dyads and to define and describe examples of:
  - Privilege
  - Discrimination
  - Oppression
  - Internalized oppression
- Discuss their answers, and offer clarifications according to the definitions (Appendix X).
- Read different scenarios from the 'D-O-P' vignettes handout (Appendix W), asking group members to identify instances of oppression, discrimination, and privilege.

Process Questions:

1. Our identities are composed of many elements (recall Session 2). How might some of our identities lead to experiences of oppression and discrimination?
   Nuestras identidades incluyen varios elementos (recordar la sesión dos). ¿Cómo podrían algunas de nuestras identidades llevarnos a experiencias de opresión y discriminación?

2. How might some identities allow us certain privileges?
   ¿Cómo pueden algunas identidades darnos ciertos privilegios?

3. Why do we discriminate?
   ¿Por qué nosotros discriminamos?

4. When are you most and least aware of your privileges?
   ¿Cuándo estás más y minímamente consciente de tus privilegios?

5. Did anything come up today that you would want to add to your shield or identities?
   ¿Surgió algo en el día de hoy que te gustaría añadir a tu escudo o identidades?

6. Did we talk about anything that related to your identity descriptor today (Session 1)?
   ¿Hablamos de algo en el día de hoy que estuviera relacionado a tus identidades (la sesión uno)?

7. Did we talk about anything that made you feel proud today? How can you use your shield to feel proud about this?
   ¿Hablamos de algo en el día de hoy que te hizo sentir orgulloso? ¿Cómo puedes usar tu escudo para sentirte orgulloso de ello?

SESSION 4: REPRESENTATION AND MISREPRESENTATION

Session Goal: To learn how certain groups are marginalized or misrepresented in society.

Time Needed: 30–45 minutes

Suggested Group Size: 3–15

Materials Needed:

- Assortment of magazines and other media materials (e.g., newspapers)
- Construction paper
- Scissors
- Glue/glue sticks
- Copies of the most recent image of the U.S. Congress

Session Directions:

- Distribute magazines, construction paper, scissors, and glue to the group members.
- Ask them to cut out pictures of people who look similar to them in terms of their various identities and to glue them onto the construction paper to create a collage.
- Have each member present their collage to the rest of the group and process. Be sure to ask questions about how easy or difficult it was to find images and how it compares with the group members' Coat of Arms and identity descriptors. Additionally, discuss how media presents images of Latino/as. Ask whether the images are realistic, inspiring, racist, sexist, insulting, etc.
- Have members look at a picture of the U.S. Congress (use the most current image).
- Process the picture. Ask them to note identities of members and missing groups. Ask them to consider the possible consequences of having only one type of leader represented.

Process Questions:

1. What is most important about today's discussion for you?
   ¿Qué fue lo más importante para ti sobre la discusión de hoy?

2. What will you take with you and use, somehow?
   ¿Qué vas a llevar contigo y poner en uso de alguna manera?

3. How will you treat others differently?
   ¿Cómo vas a tratar a otros de una manera diferente?

4. How will you ask others to treat you differently?
   ¿Cómo le pedirás a otros que te traten de una manera diferente?

5. Did anything come up today that you would want to add to your shield?
   ¿Surgió algo en el día de hoy que quisieras añadir a tu escudo?

6. Did we talk about anything that made you feel proud today? How can you use your shield to feel proud about this?
   ¿Hablamos de algo hoy que te hizo sentir orgulloso? ¿Cómo puedes usar tu escudo para sentirte orgulloso de ello?

7. How does today's session relate to social justice?
   ¿Cómo se relaciona la sesión de hoy a la justicia social?

SESSION 5: LINGUICISM

Session Goal: To explore linguicism (discrimination based on language use).

Time Needed: 30–45 minutes

Suggested Group Size: 3–15

Materials Needed:

- Copies of skit prompts for each group (Appendix Y)
- Writing utensils

Session Directions:

- Split all participants into dyads and hand each a skit prompt (Appendix Y). You can create more prompts, including ones that are most relevant to the group members' experiences or developmental levels, if desired.
- Ask participants to read the first prompt and develop a skit based on the scenarios in the prompt. Ask members to go beyond the prompt, to decide, and to practice acting out in their dyad what they think would happen next in each scenario.
- Ask each dyad to perform that first prompt for the entire group.
- Debrief each skit with the larger group before moving to the next, discussing what happened in each skit.

Process Questions:

1. Who is 'from' the United States? Who is not 'from' the United States?
   ¿Quién es 'de' los Estados Unidos? ¿Quién no es 'de' los Estados Unidos?

2. How does this relate to what language you speak? How does this relate to how you speak certain languages (accents, etc.)?
   ¿Cómo se relaciona esto al idioma que tú hablas? ¿Cómo se relaciona a como tú hablas ciertos idiomas (los acentos, etc.)?

3. Do people make assumptions about who is 'from' or 'not from' the United States based on how they look or what languages they speak? Why?
   ¿Hacen presunciones las personas sobre quién es 'de' o 'no es de' los Estados Unidos basadas en su imagen o en los idiomas que ellos hablan? ¿Por qué lo hacen?

4. What happened in today's session that was most meaningful for you?
   ¿Qué fue lo más importante para ti de la sesión del día de hoy?

5. What feelings came up for you today as we discussed this topic?
    ¿Qué emociones surgieron en el día de hoy cuando hablábamos de este tema?

6. Did we talk about anything related to your identity today?
    ¿Hablamos de algo en el día de hoy relacionado a tu identidad?

7. Did we talk about anything that made you feel proud today? How can you use your shield to be proud about this?
    ¿Hablamos de algo en el día de hoy de lo cuál te sentiste orgulloso? ¿Cómo puedes usar tu escudo para sentirte orgulloso de ello?

8. How does this session deal with social justice?
    ¿Cómo trata esta sesión con el tema de la justicia social?

SESSION 6: CRITICAL CONSCIOUSNESS AND "WHAT'S NEXT?"

Session Goal: To establish a plan for taking social justice action.

Time Needed: 30–45 minutes

Suggested Group Size: 3–15

Materials Needed:

- Handouts collected from prior sessions (if applicable)
- Writing utensils and markers/colored pencils/crayons
- Writing and construction paper
- Scissors
- Tape/glue
- Craft materials, as desired (glitter, feathers, macaroni, pipe cleaners, etc.)
- Stapler

Session Directions:

- Provide a definition of critical consciousness (e.g., the ability to critically reflect and act to change practices that maintain inequality in society). Explain how this connects to social justice, giving examples of Latino/a leaders who have enacted social justice (e.g., Cesar Chavez).
- Give each person a blank piece of paper. Ask each to write what critical consciousness means to them, and what a critically conscious world would look like in their lives.
- Ask members to draw or write examples of ways they can increase their critical consciousness or engage in social justice in their settings. Have them share.
- Provide members with two sheets of construction paper, noting the paper will be the front and back cover of their books. Allow them to decorate the paper.
- Provide members with all the handouts saved from the prior sessions.
- Have them collate their papers, add the front and back cover, and staple together.

Process Questions:

1. What is one thing you learned about yourself over the course of this group series?
   ¿Nombra una cosa que aprendiste sobre ti mismo durante el transcurso de este grupo?

2. What is one thing you learned about your peers?
    ¿Nombra una cosa que aprendiste sobre tus compañeros?

3. What is one thing you learned about the communities you live in during this group?
    ¿Nombra una cosa que aprendiste sobre las comunidades en que vives durante el transcurso del grupo?

4. Based on your experiences in this group, is there anything you would change in your Coat of Arms?
    ¿Basado en tus experiencias en este grupo, hay algo que cambiarías en tu escudo de armas?

5. Going forward, how can you contribute to social justice in the community?
    Siguiendo adelante, ¿Cómo puedes contribuir a la justicia social en la comunidad?

6. How can you make sure that you and people around you don't do things that maintain oppression and discrimination?
    ¿Cómo puedes asegurarte que tú y la gente que te rodea no hagan las cosas que mantienen la opresión y la discriminación?

Identity Definitions

Race: A social construct that groups people together according to skin tone and/or hair texture.

Raza: Una construcción social que une a un grupo de personas según el color de su piel y/o textura del cabello.

Ethnicity: A social identity that refers to shared group traits such as culture, linguistics, spirituality or religion, sociopolitical events, and traditions.

Etnicidad: Una identidad social que se refiere a las características compartidas de un grupo como la cultura, la lingüística, la espiritualidad o la religión, eventos socio-políticos, y las tradiciones.

Socioeconomic status (class): Measured by level of education, income, and occupation, but can also include the resources, prestige, and knowledge one gains from their education, income, or job.

Nivel socio-económico (clase): Se mide por el nivel de educación, ingreso, y oficio, pero también puede incluir los recursos, el prestigio, y el conocimiento que uno obtiene mediante la educación, el ingreso o un trabajo.

Ability/disability: A social identity where persons may have a mental, physical, or emotional disability. This can include a disease such as muscular atrophy or ADHD, and while some disabilities are visible (such as people who use a wheelchair), others are not. Many disabilities have a strong connection to a large community of people who suffer from the same disability, as a silent community who have their own language, culture, and customs.

Capacidad/Incapacidad: Una identidad social en la cuál una persona puede tener un impedimento físico, mental, o emocional. Esto puede incluir una enfermedad como la distrofia muscular o ADHD, y mientras algunas incapacidades son visibles (como las personas que usan una silla de rueda) otras no los son. Muchas incapacidades tienen una fuerte conexión a una gran comunidad de personas que sufren de un mismo impedimento, como la comunidad de los mudos que tiene su propio lenguaje, cultura y costumbres.

Religion: A particular system of faith and worship that influences an individual's beliefs about life's meaning, social norms, and the ultimate purpose of the universe.

Religión: Un sistema particular de fe y veneración que influye en las creencias de un individuo sobre el significado de la vida, las normas sociales, y el propósito fundamental del universo.

Assigned sex at birth: Based on primary physical sex characteristics at birth. We often think of sex as a binary with men and women on opposite sides, and that people must either be men or women. However, a person's primary or secondary sex characteristics may not neatly fit into this binary, and some do not find this binary a useful way to describe gender.

Sexo asignado al nacer: Basado en características primarias físicas presentes al nacer. A menudo pensamos del sexo como una construcción binaria, con el hombre y la mujer a lados opuestos del espectro, creyendo que las personas pueden ser hombres o mujeres. Sin embargo, las características primarias o secundarias del sexo de una persona quizás no encajen claramente entre este binario, y estas personas tal vez no encuentren este binario útil para describir su sexo.

Gender role: The role assigned to us by society/family, prescribing how we are to behave according to the sex we were assigned at birth.

Rol de género: El papel que hemos sido asignado por la sociedad/la familia, que dicta como nos debemos comportar o actuar de acuerdo al sexo que nos han asignado al nacer.

Sexual orientation: Signifies to whom we are attracted, emotionally, spiritually, and physically.

Orientación sexual: Un término que simboliza a quienes estamos atraídos emocional, espiritual, y/o físicamente.

APPENDIX V: SESSION 2: EXPLORING PRIDE AND RESILIENCY

Coat of Arms

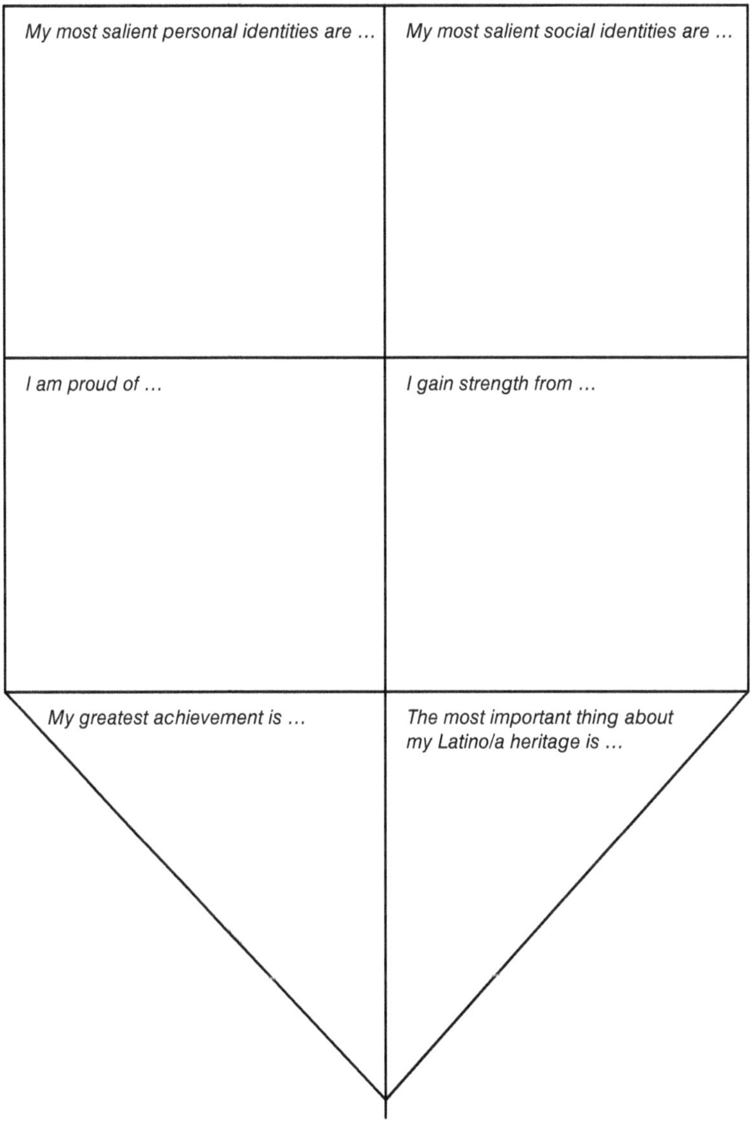

My most salient personal identities are …
My most salient social identities are …
I am proud of …
I gain strength from …
My greatest achievement is …
The most important thing about my Latino/a heritage is …

Figure 9.1 Coat of Arms

Escudo de Armas

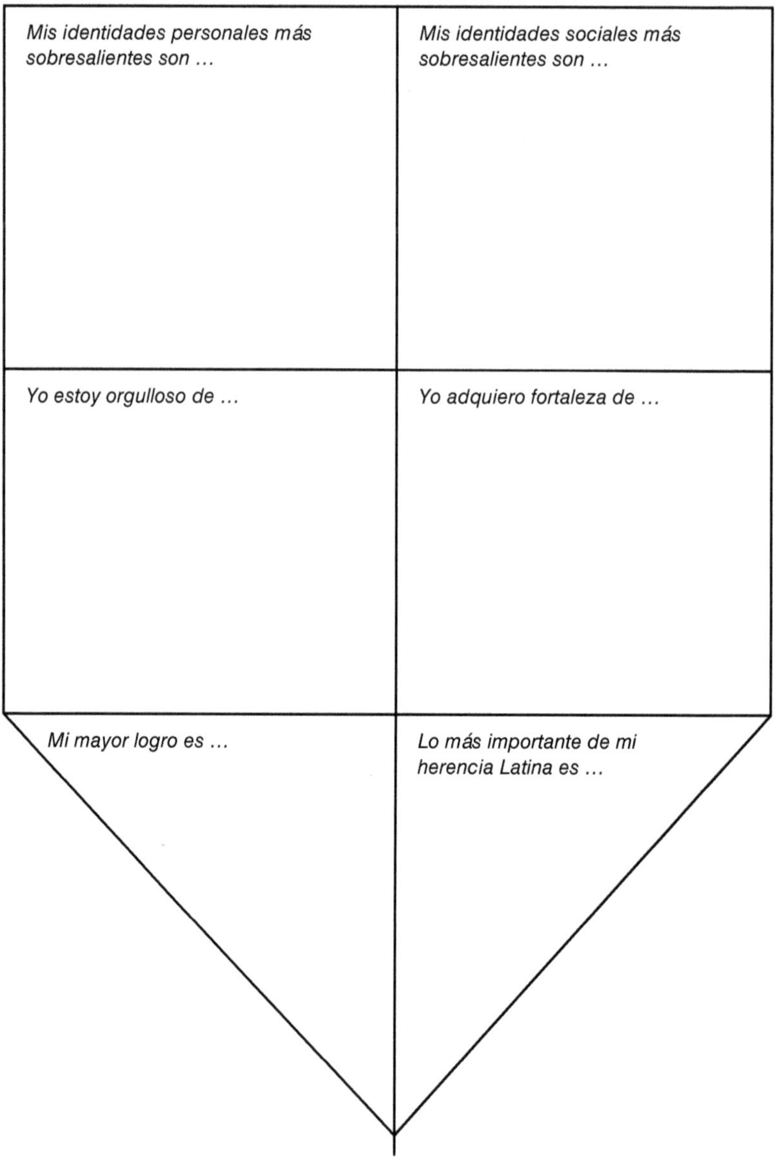

Mis identidades personales más sobresalientes son …
Mis identidades sociales más sobresalientes son …
Yo estoy orgulloso de …
Yo adquiero fortaleza de …
Mi mayor logro es …
Lo más importante de mi herencia Latina es …

Figure 9.2 Escudo de Armas

D-O-P Vignettes

Personal: Cristobal is in the lunchroom joking with some of his friends, when Cristobal's friend, James, starts doing impressions of everyone at the table. Someone asks James to do an impression of Cristobal. James laughs and says "Yo quiero Taco Bell." Everyone at the table laughs. Cristobal is embarrassed and hurt because it seems like James is making fun of his Latino identity, but doesn't say anything because he wants his friends to think he 'can take a joke.'

Personal: *Cristóbal está en la cafetería de la escuela bromeando con unos amigos, cuando uno de sus amigos, James, empieza a imitar a todos los que están sentados en la mesa. Alguien le pide a James que imite a Cristóbal. James se ríe y dice "Yo quiero Taco Bell." Todos se ríen. Cristóbal se siente avergonzado y herido porque parece que James se está burlando de su identidad Latina, pero él no le dice nada porque no quiere que sus amigos piensen que él 'no sabe tomar una broma.'*

Institutional: Adriana and her twin Marcos have played soccer since they were three years old. They recently moved to a new town and started a new high school, which has a competitive soccer team. Tryouts for the team will be held in a few weeks. Adriana and Marcos both sign up and practice for hours every day. On the day of tryouts, kids are asked to line up on the field in the order their names are listed on the coach's list. Unfortunately, while Marcos's name is on the list, Adriana's name is not. When they ask the coach why Adriana is not included, the coach tells them that the team is for "boys only."

Institucional: *Adriana y su hermano gemelo, Marcos, han jugado al fútbol desde que tenían tres años de edad. Ellos recientemente se han mudado a un nuevo pueblo y han empezado a asistir a una nueva escuela secundaria. La escuela tiene un equipo competitivo de fútbol. Las pruebas del equipo serán en unas semanas y ambos Adriana y Marcos se inscriben para intentar entrar al equipo. Ellos practican por muchas horas todos los días. El día de la prueba, se les ha pedido a todos los muchachos que se pongan en línea en el campo de fútbol en el orden de los nombres en la lista del entrenador. Desafortunadamente, el nombre de Adriana no está en la lista, pero sí el de su hermano. Cuando le preguntan al entrenador el por qué, él les dice que el equipo es solo para "varones."*

Cultural: Jazmín's family is from Puerto Rico and her family has practiced the spiritual practice of Santería for decades. Recently, Jazmín's class was given the assignment to write about an important aspect of her culture. Jazmín wrote about the importance of Santería. When she received her paper back, she saw that the teacher had given her a B. When she asked about it, he commented that Jazmín had failed to discuss the importance of Catholicism to her culture and "should have written about the actual religion practiced by most Puerto Ricans."

Cultural: La familia de Jazmín es de Puerto Rico y ha practicado la Santería por décadas. Recientemente, a Jazmín le asignaron en una de sus clases a escribir sobre un aspecto importante de su cultura. Jazmín escribió sobre la importancia de la Santería. Cuando le devolvieron su papel corregido ella notó que su profesor le había dado una B. Cuando ella le preguntó el por qué, él comentó que Jazmín no discutió la importancia del Catolicismo en su cultura y ella "debió haber escrito sobre la religión actual practicada por la mayoría de puertorriqueños."

APPENDIX X: SESSION 3: DEFINING DISCRIMINATION, OPPRESSION, AND PRIVILEGE

Definition of Classification

Discrimination: Treating someone badly because of some aspect of their identity.
Discriminación: Tratar mal a alguien debido a algún aspecto de su identidad.

Oppression: Beliefs held or acts performed that contribute to inferior treatment and/or perception of groups of people.
Opresión: La creencia o actos ejecutados que contribuyen al tratamiento inferior y/o la percepción que tenemos sobre un grupo de personas.

Internalized oppression: When the people who have experienced oppression come to believe/agree with the negative stereotypes about their group. In this way, they may possess a negative self-image due to these learned beliefs, and they may behave in a biased or oppressive way toward others from their same group.
Opresión internalizada: Cuando las personas que han sido oprimidas creen o están de acuerdo con los estereotipos negativos que existen sobre su grupo. De este modo, ellos pueden poseer una imagen propia negativa debido a las creencias que han aprendido y pueden comportarse en una manera opresiva hacia otros miembros de su mismo grupo.

Privilege: Unearned amenities, benefits, or rights accorded to a person with certain identities.
Privilegio: Servicios o beneficios inmerecidos, o derechos otorgados a una persona que posee ciertas identidades.

Nativism Skit Prompts

PROMPT #1

Sofia is in the grocery store and is in line to pay for her food. She has only recently moved to the United States and speaks very little English. Alex is the cashier and only speaks English. There is a line of customers behind Sofia, and they are in a hurry to get through the line. Create a skit of what you think could happen next in this situation.

Sofia está en la tienda de comestibles y está en línea para pagar por su comida. Ella se ha mudado recientemente a los Estados Unidos y no habla mucho inglés. Alex es el cajero y solo habla inglés. Hay una línea de clientes detrás de Sofia y ellos tienen prisa de avanzar en la línea. Crea una escena de lo que tu piensas podría pasar en esta situación.

PROMPT #2

Frankie is new to the school and does not speak English. Aaron and other students in this skit have been assigned to work in a group with Frankie. The entire group has been tasked with completing a group assignment for their class. Create a skit of what you think could happen next in this situation.

Frankie es nuevo en la escuela y no habla inglés. A Aaron y a otros estudiantes en esta escena les han asignado trabajar en un grupo con Frankie. Al grupo completo le han asignado un trabajo que tienen que completar para la clase. Crea una escena de lo que tu piensas podría pasar en esta situación.

INDEX

....

representation 153–154
resiliency 149–150, 161–162
respectful communication 135–137
respeto 8, 68
responsibility, accepting 145
role models 2, 60–61, 91
role play 64, 136
Roman Catholicism 7–8, 164

Salvadoreans 6
Santería 163–164
schools 16, 17, 21, 25; *see also* education
segregation 17, 20, 26
Selena 11
self-disclosure 42, 45
self-esteem 21, 39
self-harm 101–102
sex: assigned sex at birth 159–160;
    definition of 105
sexual orientation 90–108; coming out
    98–99, 101, 103; common vocabulary
    92–93, 103–105; constellation of stars
    90–91; definition of 105, 160; influences
    94–95; intersection of sexuality and
    ethnicity 96–97; social identities 148;
    support 100–102, 108
sexual risk taking 20
simpatía 8
Six Basic Principles of Grief 72, 84
skin color 7, 22, 40, 159
skits 155, 166
social identities 147–148, 159–160
social justice 148, 154, 156, 157–158
social supports 116–117
socioeconomic status (class) 148, 159
solidaridad 68
songs 62–63, 131–132
Sotomayor, Sonia 11
South America 6, 16
Spanish 6

stereotypes 20–21, 22, 70, 138
stories 8, 98–99; hopeful 118–119
strengths 27, 51, 55, 113
stressors and barriers 12, 15–27; career and
    educational planning 18–19; educational
    attainment 16; family acculturation
    clashes 23–24; foreign-born youth
    24–26; in-group discrimination and
    conflict 22–23; language 19; LGBTQIA
    youth 100; poverty 16–18; racial and
    ethnic discrimination 20–22; standing up
    to the bad 64–65, 70–71; teen pregnancy
    19–20
suicidality 101–102
support: grief 73; Hope Cheering Section
    116–117; LGBTQIA youth 100–102,
    108

teachers 17, 21
team work 54
teen pregnancy 19–20
Texas 6
Tijerina, Reies López 10
traditions 7–9, 27, 36, 43
transgender, definition of 105
transsexuals 105
trauma 18, 24

undocumented immigrants 25–26
unemployment 16

values 7–8, 27; counselor's identity 43;
    ethnic identity 36; grief 73; values tree
    58–59, 68–69
violence 17

Wade, Dwayne 124
Whiteness 40
willpower thinking 110, 122
words of wisdom 82–83

For Product Safety Concerns and Information please contact our EU
representative GPSR@taylorandfrancis.com
Taylor & Francis Verlag GmbH, Kaufingerstraße 24, 80331 München, Germany

www.ingramcontent.com/pod-product-compliance
Ingram Content Group UK Ltd.
Pitfield, Milton Keynes, MK11 3LW, UK
UKHW021056080625
459435UK00003B/26